WAKE UP
TO YOUR
WEIGHT LOSS

Using the Art of Personal Narrative to
Achieve Your Best Body

ALYSON MEAD

A STORIED LIFE
New York • Los Angeles

Library of Congress Cataloging-In-Publication Data

Mead, Alyson
Wake up to your weight loss / by Alyson Mead — 1st US ed.

p. cm.
1. Health & Fitness – Weight Loss   2. Self Help – Weight Loss
3. Meditation—Spirituality   4. Writing—How To

PRINTED IN THE UNITED STATES OF AMERICA

First U.S. Edition: May 2008

EAN 13: 9781427611000

Book design by James Arneson

First Printing

For Emily

CONTENTS

Introduction

When we want to say that someone is serious or dignified, we say she has *gravitas*, meaning substance. When we believe someone's opinion to be important, influential or authoritative, we say his words "carry great weight."

So when did weight become synonymous with fat, lazy and dissolute?

Our obsession with weight has not been confined to the last century, though the advent of mass advertising and constant barrage of media messages may suggest otherwise. Every day of our lives, we see and hear millions of verbal and non-verbal cues, around which we orient our behavior, and our emotional responses, relative to our bodies. Let's face it — the overwhelming majority of people we see, in print ads and on television, are much thinner than the norm. We see these people leading happy lives, to which we all aspire. And after seeing or hearing the message repeatedly, we internalize it, making it seem as if these are the individuals who deserve our attention and, most of all, our love.

Despite all this, we continue to become heavier and heavier as a society. Currently, Americans are dangerously overweight, with more than 3.8 million people weighing 300 pounds or more. Another 400,000 people, mostly men, weigh over 400 pounds.

Additionally, the National Center for Health Statistics and the Centers for Disease Control's BMI (Body Mass Index) statistics indicate that 63% of Americans are overweight, and 31% are obese. Only 1 in 5 adults fall within our currently prescribed weight charts. At the same time, childhood obesity is increasing at alarming rates, having more than tripled in the past two decades.

How can this happen? We are a prosperous, information-filled society, in which most people have access to advanced medical care and adequate nutrition. Why do we not heed the warnings? According to a recent U.S. Surgeon General's Report, 100,000 deaths occur each year as a result of obesity. Carrying extra weight puts us at greater risk for heart attacks and stroke, cancer, cardiovascular disease and diabetes.

Sometimes, it seems, we try to take more control. The National Institute of Health Statistics estimates that "diet-conscious adults" will increase by 50% this year. And in 2003:

- 65% of U.S. citizens tried some form of weight loss or weight control.
- 49% attempted to lose at least five pounds.
- 16% attempted to maintain their weight.

Only 20% of these people were "very" or "extremely" successful, though. Why?

The New England Journal of Medicine tells us that losing even a small amount of excess body weight can help decrease our risk of disease, and positively affect our longevity. We listen, but halfway, it appears, spending a great deal of money (around $38 billion last year) in an effort to lose weight, without achieving much success.

෴

Like many people, I have struggled with weight issues. I first become aware of my size, relative to that of other kids, in first grade. I was six years old when all the students in my class had to line up along the blackboard, from shortest to tallest. I'm sure there was a lesson in there somewhere, but all I remember was feeling mortified that I was taller than all but one of the boys, and that the prettiest, most popular little girls fell decidedly towards the shorter end of the range.

I attempted my first diet at ten years old, after a boy called me fat on the playground. Without telling my mother, I began to skip meals, usually breakfast, which I'd never had much use for anyway. By lunch-time, I'd be seeing silvery sparkles whirling around in my field of vision. It became hard to focus on my schoolwork, and I often held my breath to keep from fainting in class.

By the time I was an adolescent, shy and still tall, I had begun reading fashion magazines, like *Seventeen* and *Glamour*, and found out that most models were my size (5' 9") and weighed about 125 pounds. No wonder that boy had called me fat! At 155 pounds, I had my work cut out for me. For the duration of junior high, I skipped both breakfast *and* lunch, and played tennis with my friends during our lunch break. I was proud of myself for killing two birds with one stone—no food and taking part in a calorie-burning activity—*genius*!

In high school, a friend told me about diet pills. Once I started working, first as a baby sitter and then as an attendant at a local beach, I made this purchase part of my weekly ritual: cash paycheck, go to drugstore, get diet pills, wash two down in the parking lot with a caffeine-laced Tab. Then get on with life, feeling skinnier and more desirable already.

I lost weight—a lot of it. Within a few weeks, none of my clothes fit, and I was down to 132 on the bathroom scale. I figured that by the time summer rolled around, I would be at "modeling weight," though I had no real plans to model.

My first surprise was that boys came hurtling out of the woodwork. The popular, sulky ones, who'd never given me the time of day before, hung around my locker or pushed notes at me in study hall. I never had to walk alone in the halls. Instead, there was always someone handy to carry my books or drive me home from school, Led Zeppelin blasting out the Trans-Am windows.

It was so obvious, I thought: less weight really did equal more popularity. I gave it a formula, doodling in my calculus notebook:

$$-W = P^{10}$$
(Where W is weight and P is popularity)

I doubted there were major scientific prizes for this sort of thing, but it kept me from being bored during class.

Maintaining my weight loss wasn't hard, as long as I never ate, which started to be no problem at all. Cravings for food were pushed aside by other concerns. Everyone in my family has always been pretty athletic, so I played sports during both seasons of the school year: tennis in the fall, and volleyball in the spring.

The diet pills and steady diet of caffeinated soda kept me going all the way through a long school day and an hour and a half of after-school practice. But though my heart raced and my veins pulsed with extra energy all day, I started getting incredibly tired before 4:30, when practice ended. I relied more and more on the asthma inhalers I'd grown up with (as emergency measures) in order to finish the day, and never even considered eating anything more substantial than an apple. No one interfered; no one even knew.

Soon, the "sparkles," as I called them, were part of my everyday experience. I saw them when I woke up in the morning, when I stood up suddenly, and felt the queasy, fast-dropping jolt of dizziness, and when I tried to concentrate on the blackboard during my classes. All the caffeine coursing through my body, along with the over-the-counter speed, prevented me from sleeping at night. Each night, I lay awake in a slash of moonlight, counting the number of times my heart could beat each minute.

I continued playing sports, attending classes, going to parties and dating, though my mind was always on my appearance. How did I look to others? Did they really like me? Or was that other girl, the thinner one, more worthy of attention?

When I attended family functions, I pushed the food around on my plate, too mortified to let anyone witness my eating. I waved the waitress back to the table several times during each meal for more water, until everyone commented that I must have diabetes or something. Over time, I grew thinner and thinner. Everyone said that with my looks, I really should think about modeling.

The insane yo-yo dieting and copious ingestion of speed continued through college, though now the speed came in handy as a way to stay up longer, in order to cram for exams. Diet Coke replaced Tab as the drink of choice for most of the young women I knew, and we drank so much of it, we got terrible headaches in the morning if we didn't crack open a can within a few seconds of opening our eyes. Often, I carried one can to my earliest class, and had another stashed in my backpack for a late morning pick-me-up. I stopped playing sports, and started going to lots of foreign films and art galleries. Fitness became uncool. Other things became a lot more important.

As luck would have it, I was led back to fitness for the same reason I had originally taken it up—heartbreak and confusion. It was a few years past graduate school and I was in an almost five-year long relationship that really wasn't going anywhere, but causing me pain so constant I had to push it away in my mind just so I could keep functioning in my job. After I broke it off, I felt more isolated than ever before. My friends were his friends; I had made very few of my own in New York. And he was everywhere I was likely to go, since we lived and worked in close proximity to one another.

Change was crucial. I got myself a new apartment, even though I had never lived alone before, and a new gym membership. I spoke with a trainer about working together, and soon I counted myself among the people who made trips to the gym five times or more each week, just to feel good about myself.

I lost the weight I had regained by being miserable in my relationship, and even a few additional pounds. At that point, I was the thinnest I had been since high school. And, just as before, guys surfaced, wanting whatever they wanted from me. After thirty years of being there for everyone but myself, though, a relationship was the last thing on my mind.

That time was among the most painful in my life. But it began the process of returning to myself and, ultimately, of returning to my body.

Ask anyone in my family and they're likely to tell you that I've always been a curious person. I enjoy reading, and can't imagine my life without a stack of books next to my bed. The subject matter seldom matters. What's important is that a compelling question is answered, or that an unclear image—of a culture, place, or concept—has been clarified.

At that moment in my life, the question that needed clarifying was my health, and the relationship of my mind and emotional life to my physical body. Sure, I was capable of consuming fewer calories and burning more of them, but did that mean I truly understood the complicated relationships between my body, mind and spirit?

I didn't think so.

I started reading everything I could—about the relationship between asthma inhalers and weight gain, caffeine, pollution, herbs— anything that might be able to help me work with my body, instead of against it. At the same time, I began to take the yoga classes offered through my gym, and explore the practices of Ayurvedic, Chinese and Tibetan medicine.

I stopped taking anything stronger than aspirin, and that only when a headache got so bad I couldn't stand it. I quit drinking diet sodas, enduring four days of crushing headaches and equally sleepless nights. Finally, I started eating as many whole grains and fresh fruits and vegetables as I could, leaving out red meat and substituting other protein sources.

There were many temptations, but as I worked with my mind and body together, during yoga classes, I realized that I had never been encouraged to think of them as related. The body was a disconnected thing that was to be shoved about and manipulated as I (or whomever I was currently allowing to make that decision for me) saw fit. My mind was separate and rational, like a scientist conducting an experiment. All along, I had not been treating myself as a wholly integrated person, but as a sort of human lab rat, to be dissected, used and exploited.

Shortly thereafter, I moved to California, and found a support-ive atmosphere for alternative spirituality and medicine. Exercising became fully integrated into my life, as did shopping at farmer's markets for locally cultivated fruits and vegetables. All was well, until I started feeling dead tired before it was time for dinner.

I have always been a very active person. My family members still tease me about reading books while listening to music and having the television on, or about the sheer number of tasks I can take on (and accomplish) in record time. So feeling not just beat but bone-tired before the end of my workday was really terrifying. At the same time, weight began to creep back onto my frame, though my eating and exercising habits hadn't changed.

At first, I chalked it up to a toxic and unsupportive workplace. Maybe I had been overeating, and needed to exercise more. My husband (then my boyfriend) and I arranged to go on more hikes. I ate salads every day, but the weight wouldn't come off. I bought larger clothing and stopped looking in mirrors. I told myself it was temporary, that it would all be over soon. It was as if I were trapped in a dream, and could will myself awake.

By accident, I was diagnosed with having an underactive thyroid. My physician had just finished lecturing me about being overweight, telling me to stop eating at McDonald's (which I never did), when she asked off-handedly, "Has anyone ever tested your thyroid?"

They had not. I went for a blood test and found that my TSH (Thyroid Stimulating Hormone) was the highest my doctor had ever seen. Her assistant left me a message saying they had called in a prescription for a popular drug designed to lower this number, but would not return my calls when I wanted to ask about other options (or even what that number meant in the scheme of her diagnosis). I never picked up that prescription, and changed doctors after a week of unreturned phone calls.

Again, I devoted myself to reading, trolling the Internet for forums and chat rooms, poring over countless articles, scientific papers, and books. I even bought a copy of the *Physicians' Desk Reference*, so I could learn what the drug my old doctor had prescribed, or any of the others, might do to my body in the long run.

On the Internet, I found a very large and devoted community of people dealing with thyroid issues. Names of "understanding" doctors were exchanged, as well as information on new drug and lifestyle studies. Many others had been treated the same way I had, by a dismissive doctor who clearly didn't have time to treat overweight people. Perhaps he or she assumed we were all lazy, and had clearly brought the problem on ourselves.

The process really opened my eyes. When we are alone, and trying to measure ourselves against what our culture deems attractive, it's easy to get downhearted or even hopeless about the prospect of being thin, or achieving a healthy weight. Now I saw that thyroid disorders were considered a "woman's problem," and were addressed with the same kind of dismissive treatment that migraine headaches and Pre-Menstrual

Syndrome used to be, when women were labeled "hysterics." I tried to find out how many people, not just women, were affected by this condition, but the information was not widely available. I wondered if there were other conditions like it, adding additional weight to our frames without being accompanied by increased eating.

Trying to strike a compromise, I spoke to my new doctor about what I had found, and tried to factor his expertise into my decision-making process. But when my endocrinologist told me that it was nearly impossible to lose the weight I had gained, not because of my lowered metabolic rate but because I was over 40, I took it as a direct challenge. Over the next year, I devoted myself to learning as much as I could about how the human body develops and stores weight. I read books by experts, ingested scientific papers on physiognomy, and attended talks by spiritual teachers who made parallels between weight, stress and emotional turmoil.

Though my new thyroid hormone supplements took some time to "work," and I was only marginally less tired, I began to work out again, walking as long as I could on a treadmill and then stopping, or going for an easy hike. Eventually, I added more challenging exercises, and began to feel stronger at my core.

At the same time, I refused to treat my body with any further disrespect. I vowed not to go on any starvation diets, have risky surgery, or take any sort of drug. I ate normal portions of balanced meals, with as much fresh, local produce as I had access to at that time of year. After a few weeks, my body started to feel different inside. Lightness and strength began to co-exist, almost like the sun breaking through clouds. Then my body started to shed the weight it no longer needed.

So far I have lost ninety pounds, and I'm waiting for my body to tell me where its healthiest weight lies. I have vowed to work with my body no matter where it wants to stop, because for the first time in my life, I have begun to trust this place that houses my soul. I'm still here to tell the tale, and a lot healthier for it.

I wanted to write this book for everyone who's ever struggled with his or her weight, especially if you've ever had moments of hating your body. When you think about it, what a strange concept that is.

Our Creator of choice gives us a home, to protect our organs and soul, and we turn it into a forum for self-hatred and psychodrama.

I don't believe that our natural state is self-hatred, nor do I believe that any real change is possible while under its spell. But though new diet books flood the marketplace every year few, if any, deal with the emotional repercussions of added weight, or the sometimes harrowing emotional journey required to bring one's body into balance.

In the time I devoted to learning more about the way my body stored and lost weight, I started a storytelling practice like the one I'd developed in my first book, *Wake Up to Your Stories*. This time, though, I focused on issues surrounding weight, size and self-image. The exercises and meditations in this book are the result of that practice.

I believe there are many more reasons why people hold onto weight than just the calories they consume versus the calories they burn. But with that being said, I am not a medical doctor (maybe in my next life!), and this book is not meant to take the place of a doctor's advice in your life. If you plan to undertake any sort of diet and exercise plan, it's always best to make an appointment to talk with your doctor or health care practitioner, to make sure your desired path is a safe one.

Wake Up to Your Weight Loss is a program designed to accompany any food and exercise plan, and offer the emotional and spiritual support that's usually lacking. When I was obsessed with my body image as a younger person, there was no way to check myself against a healthy looking person, or a healthy *feeling* person, for that matter. All that mattered was the outside, the wrapping. Today, some of us are still taught that the body is somehow outside us, and as long as we follow steps X, Y and Z, our desired results will appear.

It may sound obvious, but our bodies are part of us, and we are part of our bodies. We *are* our bodies, just as they are us. Separating our bodies from the mind and spirit only reinforces a negative self-opinion, and keeps us from enjoying the fullest fruits of a wonderful, mystifying and surprising existence on this planet.

This program is designed to take place over a period of nine weeks, with each chapter, along with its meditations and exercises, pertaining to emotional issues that tend to come up while trying to lose weight. If you want to condense this program into a smaller time frame, that's fine, too. Or you can expand the program as well, by taking 2-3 weeks or more to experience the exercises in each chapter.

Lastly, you are free to pick and choose the issues that may be affecting you the most. I have found, in exploring this program with others, that it's best to move through the chapters in order. But if you're suffering, and could find relief in practicing a chapter towards the end of the book, please feel free to do so.

Some of my readers have found that forming a small group, and going through the meditations and follow-up exercises together, is helpful as well. Since added weight sometimes makes us invisible to others, the act of bearing witness, hearing the stories of others, and being heard in turn, can be a very powerful tool to help support your weight loss program.

The main thing to remember, when starting this type of program, is that you are not alone. There are millions of people just like you, all over the globe, struggling with how they want their bodies to look and feel, and how they want to relate to themselves as a wholly integrated human being. We are remarkably resilient, and are truly here to help one another make it through.

Chapter One

How Can a Storytelling Practice Help?

We are, no matter where we come from, or how we engage with the dominant culture, constantly surrounded by stories. As infants, before we even know what words are, we are told stories. These stories help us dispel fear before we go to sleep, learn morals and other societal values, and even establish a connection with our caretakers.

From the time we're at our smallest and most vulnerable, stories are the glue that binds us to others like us. Researchers have found that infants are incredible sponges for information, reading the slightest changes in inflection, facial expression and body language. The same is true for the way we experience stories. Even as adults, we can hear a gripping story and become completely lost, projecting ourselves into the story and feeling all the emotions as if they were our own. Today, "reality" television picks up some of the slack from that phenomenon, allowing us to have love affairs, heal a problem, or go on an amazing adventure, all within an hour-long timeslot.

Children often need stories in order to figure out the complex emotional world of adults. Remember hiding out in a tree or other out-of-the-way place, making up stories with your friends? Remember how doing that made it seem like you were in charge of your world, even if that wasn't technically true?

As we grow and develop, though, we leave our stories behind. Kids are always in a hurry to be a fourth grader, or a seventh grader, or a se-

13

nior in high school. They want whatever's cool, hip, dangerous or seemingly grown up. Often, this doesn't include creating and sharing stories, especially if it involves spending any more time with their parents.

But just as we leave our homes, at eighteen, if we decide to get a job, or after college, we need our stories most of all. We need something familiar, which will help us make this brand new transition in our lives, and we need something that's uniquely ours, so we can keep developing our sense of self. It is the sense of self that will carry us towards our goals, whether they're personal or professional in nature.

Our stories, then, perform three major functions for us:

• Our stories are the connective tissue that reminds us to be human.
• Our stories provide our memory, foundation and "moral compass."
• Our stories protect us from the lowest aspects of our own nature.

It is at this time of our lives, when everything is changing, that we have to make some quick decisions about the kind of people we'll allow ourselves to become. What will become most important: love, money, family or spirituality? If we want a weekend out with friends, is it all right to pay the rent late? And what if the person we love doesn't love us back?

Stories are one important tool we have to deal with major transitions. But keeping a diary or blog may not work for everyone. Many of my students have said the act of keeping a diary feels like shouting into the void, or as if no one is really listening. Personally, every time I try to keep one, I feel like the most boring person on earth.

So where's a person to start?

A Brief History of Storytelling

Human beings started to keep records of their existence from the beginning of history as we currently understand it. We can only guess that they needed a way to explain the world around them, and to leave behind a record of their experience. No one knows for sure why they did this, especially when issues of survival were so pressing.

The stories of early civilizations often centered around the search for food, including the killing of animals, and the gathering and storing of other foodstuffs. Other important topics were the family structure, especially as it related to the distribution of power and responsibility, and the building of communities. Establishing security became a primary concern, and any immediate threats to their survival, such as inclement weather or predators, were immediately dispatched with sacrifices, ritual or song.

Likewise, tribes lauded a successful hunt by praising their gods and/or goddesses with elaborate ceremonies designed to curry favor. Other stories sent tribal members into the afterlife, by reaffirming the culture's burial methods and remembering the deceased's life as it had been on earth.

Other legacies of early storytelling can be found in some of the Old Stone Age (30,000 BCE - 10,000 BCE) caves, particularly those in Lascaux and Chauvet, France. Inhabitants of the caves used soil, crushed rocks and plants to make natural pigments, and used sticks and other implements to apply them directly onto the walls of the caves.

In one cave, a racing herd of animals can be seen (these are thought to be horses or red deer), along with geometric designs that some believe stand in for the phases of the sun and/or moon. A series of large dots, a semicircle of smaller dots, a V-shaped bat like symbol—no one knows for sure what these meant to the original cave-dwellers.

What is most touching about the cave paintings of Lascaux and Chauvet are the red silhouettes of human hands. These appear to have been made by blowing or spraying pigment over the artist's hand, and are present in almost all of the ancient caves. When I look at the pictures of these hands, it's easy to connect with the fact that there was a person on the other end of this experience, and that he or she was trying to be seen, across millennia, just as you or I do today.

The Five Reasons We Need Stories

In studying how stories have been told over the years, I have found that there are five main reasons we need stories in our lives:

- An Explanation of the World Around Us
- A Way to Honor the Supernatural
- A Way to Entertain Ourselves
- A Way to Gain Immortality, by Connecting with Our Ancestors
- A Way to Express the Beauty of Human Existence

Each of these reasons corresponds with a deeper need within us—to be seen and heard, to understand the mysterious, to play, connect and express ourselves. And many of these needs often go unmet in our daily lives, whether we're trying to lose weight or not.

Our experience with stories began when we were very emotionally pliable. Our brains were developing, and we were at our most receptive, simply so we could survive. But that way of experiencing stories doesn't seem to change all that much as we age. Even today, stories are able to get deeper into our consciousness than other methods of communication. Just as beautiful music sometimes penetrates the way we see, engendering powerful emotional responses while bypassing any emotional guard we may have constructed, stories can trigger very old responses that may have been stored in the mind, or even in the tissues of the body, from the time we were children.

We do not cease to need stories when we pass a certain age, or when society decides we're adults. Even if we're working at a job, engaging in a creative project, or raising a family, we need our stories to help us make important decisions.

After all, what is "Cinderella" but a manual for finding and dating the right man?

What is "Snow White" but a cautionary tale about jealousy?

What is the story of King Solomon but an illustration of true parental love?

And what is "The Emperor's New Clothes" but a lesson in telling the truth?

Identifying your own stories, and developing a practice that allows you to tell them on a regular basis, can help you learn more about yourself and your true feelings in a safe way (this can especially apply if your true feelings are undesirable in nature, since we tend to want to disown these). Additionally, incorporating a storytelling practice in your life can help you discover reasons you may be holding onto excess weight, and reveal unique, internal strategies to help you realize your weight loss goals. Lastly, this practice can help build confidence, and help dispel false messages that may have already been internalized by living within a narrow cultural definition of beauty.

The Six Ways We Use Stories

Along with the five ways we need stories, there are also six ways we tend to use stories in our daily lives:

- Healing from Abuse or Neglect
- Connecting with Relatives and Family Members
- To Leave Something Behind
- To Express Ourselves and the World We Live In
- To Become More Visible
- To Ensure That Our Way of Life Continues

Establishing that we need stories in our lives, to help us recognize and achieve our goals, as well as dispel any obstacles that may reside inside us, is one thing. But in order to create a storytelling practice that can help us achieve real results, we will need to look into how we're already using stories in our day-to-day lives.

All of us do it. We come home from work, shuck off our coat and put down our purse or briefcase. Then we talk to our mates, friends, children or roommates about the events of our days: the triumphs and the painful parts, the irritations and moments of excitement and joy. In essence, we are telling the story of our day, embellishing it with different voices, if we had a fight with the guy at the post office, or funny asides, to illustrate what might have been going through our minds at a particular moment. Unconsciously, we use these stories all the time.

We may be trying to convert someone to our way of seeing things, if we've had an argument, or to garner support, if we've had a bad day. We may be trying to prove a point, if we feel righteous about a wrong that has been committed, or even draw ourselves closer to someone, if we can share a similar tale that's happened to us.

The bottom line is that stories are part of our lives on a moment-to-moment basis. All you have to do is recognize that you have them, and that you're already using them. Once that happens, you can learn to channel this power towards whatever you want to achieve. For example, if you're always fighting with people, from the guy at the post office to the people in your family, you may wish to look at how you're "storytelling" about anger. If you're always complaining about having to take on more work than you're comfortable doing, you might look into your "storytelling" on fear or duty.

This is more complicated than simply thinking about it, or even writing about it in a journal. Creating and nurturing a storytelling practice demands nothing less than your devotion to reach inside yourself, sometimes to your deepest, softest places, in order to pull out the darkest, richest material. This can help make your writing deeper, if you're already engaged with this discipline. But it can also help you adopt coping strategies for common or uncommon problems, and develop confidence to take action wherever it's required. Your storytelling practice can be as unique and varied as you are, adapting to the myriad changes of your days, reflecting and revealing by turns.

Why Meditation?

Eastern spirituality was introduced to the West in the late 1950s, through Beat writers and poets like Jack Kerouac and Allen Ginsberg, and furthered in the 1960s, with the influx of teachers like Chogyam Trungpa Rinpoche and Thich Nhat Hanh, originally trained in Asia. Westerners are still sorting out the effects of these ancient practices on a world more attuned to the Big Gulp than the Heart Sutra.

Meditation, an integral part of practice for Buddhists, Hindus, and other Eastern religions, is a practice which helps to train the mind away from its busyness, as well as its tendency to run away with us sometimes. If you've ever sat in meditation for any length of time, you may have begun to notice that your mind tends to dart way from you, retelling a story that has already happened, becoming lost in fantasy, or moving forward, into a story you have yet to live. Your mind may also take you in a mundane direction, telling the story of what you'll have for dinner, or how you'll cope with a work challenge later this week. It seems that no matter where we live on the planet, our human minds need to think. Maybe Descartes was right when he said, "I think, therefore I am."

Because meditation works with the mind, and most writing comes from this same source, they seem to share the same, if not a very similar, process. I believe that humans simply cannot exist without our stories, and that stories are as much part of our physiology as our digestive or respiratory systems.

However, storytelling is not just a mental activity. Though it seems to originate in the mind, and our minds seem to want to embellish our stories with very little provocation, our stories sometimes lodge themselves into the tissues of the body, only to become stuck there, until they are dislodged by trauma, exercise or bodywork like massage, shiatsu or rolfing. Scientists such as Candace Pert, who has been studying the relationship between the mind and body for close to three decades, have found that we are hard-wired for bliss, literally, by the molecules comprising our bodies.

So meditation is a very important part of any storytelling practice. With meditation, we can get beyond our mental and emotional "walls," which have been erected to keep us from moving toward the slimy, scary stuff in our own natures. You may have had this experience—I know I've had it many times. You pick up a book and start reading. The prose is perfect. Every word feels as if it's been there forever, carved in stone, and couldn't be replaced with any other words, ever. It's amazing, and you're in awe of this author's talent, so much so that you never notice that you're not drawn into the story at all. It's as if the author is ignoring you completely, and whatever you might get out of the book. He or she exists in an untouchable little shell. And you don't matter at all.

I call this Airless Prose, and all writers, professional or not, can fall into this trap. We all love to be thought of as clever and talented, and many of us can fall in love with the talent we've been given, or have developed on our own. What makes this possible is an over-concentration on the mental aspects of storytelling, to the detriment of its physical effects.

You do not have to have a tough and masculine prose style like Ernest Hemingway to begin telling stories with your body as well as your mind. You merely have to understand and accept that there is an unbreakable connection between these two aspects of your self, and strive to find ways to help them communicate more effectively.

How Meditation Works

Over the past two decades, the Dalai Lama has met with some of the best scientific minds in the West to discuss the ways in which his native Buddhist practice overlaps with the pursuits of science. Over the course of several days, in formal talks and informal dialogues, the people behind the Mind-Life Conference group try to get at the intersection of science and faith, and the space where one may in fact influence and inform the other.

One fascinating outcome of this ongoing dialogue is that scientists have been able to observe the vital statistics of various subjects while they're meditating, in order to measure changes to the brain, and to the neurological system that supports its functioning. This important work continues each year through the Mind and Life Institute, in Boulder, Colorado, and its programs throughout the world.

There are several kinds of meditation, used for many secular and religious reasons. *Shamatha vipassana*, also called "insight" or "clear seeing" meditation is one style used widely to tame the mind (more on that in a minute). *Shamatha* is a Sanskrit word which means to bring about calmness in the mind and body. *Vipassana* adds heightened awareness and sensitivity, either to the object of meditation, or to the world at large.

Some people equate meditation with "blissing out," or simply letting go of the petty concerns that drive all of our lives at one time or another. That can be one benefit of meditation, as well as its various properties of stress relief. But meditation is an important tool not just for physical and mental relaxation, but to help us become more sensitive and aware as humans, and as storytellers writing our own lives. This storytelling can be done on paper, using a computer, or become the fodder for our thoughts and actions as we exist from day to day. The same process can also be indispensable when considering or attempting a program of exercise and/or weight loss.

During meditation, there are subtle and not-so-subtle changes that occur in the mind and body. First, as the breath comes more slowly and the heart rate slows in response, the metabolism slows down. Long-time meditators often report needing to sleep less, eat less and even breathe less because of their practice. The normal rate of breathing for most people, for example, is 15-16 times per minute. While meditating, some have reported breathing only two or three times per minute.

As well, brainwaves begin to increase, especially in the alpha frequencies of 8-12 cycles per second. This process usually does not occur whenever we have our eyes open and are concentrating on the details of our conscious lives. Additionally, the muscles relax, the sympathetic nervous system is depressed, blood pressure drops, and brain chemistry is altered.

If these physiological changes are combined with a conscious method of focusing, we begin to see changes in the way our minds receive and process information, as well as the way we feel about the information received, and then how we choose to react to it. This process is often referred to as "taming the mind."

Taming the mind begins with adopting a posture of meditation (we will get to this shortly) and either focusing on a particular goal or exercise (a guided meditation) or using a focusing device, such as a mantra, chant, or even a phrase or affirmation. The type of meditation we'll use in this book asks that whenever you find yourself having a thought, or getting carried away in a storyline, that you bring yourself back to the present moment by saying "thinking" to yourself. The goal is not to wipe the mind clean, or to stop yourself from having thoughts. Instead, it is to become familiar with the fact that we are all constantly writing stories in our minds. Thoughts are the building blocks of these storylines. Labeling thoughts lets us know that we're noticing them for what they are, and not getting carried away by them in an unconscious way.

Sometimes, our storylines can take us in a positive direction. When we set goals, for example, or aspire to reach certain heights in our creative endeavors, we're using stories to spur us on. These stories can also take us in negative directions, by reminding us how clumsy, inefficient, or fat we are, to the detriment of our self-image.

Certain scientists, such as Dr. James Austin, have even suggested that meditation can literally rewire the circuitry of the brain. In his book *Zen and the Brain* (Austin, 1999), he details the results of MRI tests given to meditators, and charting the ever-changing electrical information inside their brains. For instance, the act of exhaling, which we do approximately half of the time, helps quiet the brain, according to EEG results.

All the data suggest that meditation, when combined with action and lifestyle changes, can result in the transformation of the physiological body. But anyone who has ever been on a diet knows that once the diet is stopped, the pounds creep back on. To me, this thinking suggests a profound disconnect between the mind and its desires, and the body and its needs. I have found, in working with myself and others, that only when "head" exercises like meditation are followed up with "body" experiences, by taking your meditation practice off the mat, can real and lasting change occur.

The second main challenge I have heard from dieters is that they often feel alone, or without support. Groups like Weight Watchers have tried to alleviate some of this loneliness by hosting weekly meetings, in which members can ask questions or get to know each other. Many find that the process of losing weight is easier when done with a friend.

But though this may be helpful for some, it often does not address the central issue of loneliness within us. Being overweight is lonely. Weight sometimes stands, literally, between you and the people you want to know better. I have spoken with people who literally feel lost inside the bulk of their bodies. That kind of deep, inner loneliness can only be addressed by looking inside, working with the mind, and then taking the practice off the mat in order to interact with others. This extends the practice beyond itself, and cements the connections among all creatures, regardless of whether they're trying to lose weight or not. The stigma of carrying extra weight is often decreased as well. Confidence and strength can grow from there, and each person can forge his or her individual path toward fulfillment.

How the Program Works

Wake Up to Your Weight Loss is a program designed to take place over the course of nine weeks. No matter if you'll be on a diet for one week or two years, or even if you choose not to diet at all, the lessons, meditations and follow-up exercises in each chapter are meant to represent one stage of the internal weight loss journey, which I believe will support and foster your continued success. Each chapter is meant to be read and worked with over the course of a week, though if you plan on trying to change your body for a longer period of time, they can be adapted. You may choose to work with Chapter 1 for two weeks, for example, or even three months. As long as it's helping you create a stronger and more intentional link between your mind and body, there's no wrong way to do this.

Each chapter will discuss one very potent emotional issue that has tended to come up for the people I've worked with, myself included.

Though most diet books are wonderful at giving instructions for how many calories to eat, or how often to exercise, few, if any, delve into the very real emotional transitions losing weight can entail. These can be fear, at being seen for who you are for the very first time, or anger, at being ignored because of extra weight, or something else entirely.

Again, this book is not meant to take the place of a physician or a fitness trainer. It's always best to check in with your chosen professional to help you in those areas. *Wake Up to Your Weight Loss* already assumes that you have the tools you need to succeed. In working with your mind as you lose weight, you may find that you are far better prepared to weather the internal and external changes ahead.

What You Need

Since each chapter will present a brief "talk," or lesson, a meditation, and then two follow-up exercises, you will need very few things to complete this program. The first is a notebook and a writing implement of some kind. If you do not consider yourself a writer, or are prevented from writing for some reason, you are free to record your thoughts and experiences using a mini-cassette recorder, which can usually be had for about $35 from an electronics store.

The second thing you will need is a space to call your own, preferably in your home. If you meditate already, you may have invested in a cushion. But if not, it's important to start with claiming a space for yourself, especially if you live with others. It's too easy to allow important goals like weight loss, along with better care and nurturance of your body, to get lost in the shuffle when co-existing with your job, relationships, home life and other commitments. Finding a place you will return to every day to meditate and practice the exercises in this book will, over time, convince you that you are worth the time, effort and even space it will take to reinforce the connection between your mind and body.

In order to complete the program, you will also need the sincere desire to work with whatever comes up for you, whether it be painful or joyful, frustrating or mundane. The mistaken belief about meditation is that it is somehow magical, bestowing peace and light on whomever it touches. But meditation is simply a tool, to help you focus in on and, more importantly, learn to cope with the stuff your mind may fling at you.

This program requires attention, and effort, and the willingness to be authentic. It's not about finding just the positive things, while leaving the negative behind. Sometimes, our lives are just not that simple. Negative emotions can be tempered. Negative experiences can be processed and released. But that does not mean that they can be permanently removed from your life. These exercises provide one way to cope in a way that doesn't let negativity weigh you down, no pun intended. Though none of us can control what may come about in the future, we can develop tools to help us deal with the natural ebb and flow of life.

With that being said, *Wake Up to Your Weight Loss* is a program that grew out of my deep love for people of all sizes, and the strange, wonderful things they do and say. I believe that every single living being has at least one story, and can benefit from writing or speaking it out loud, and sharing it with others. If you are willing to devote a small part of your day each day to working with your mind, and trying to take what you have learned into your "real" life, I believe you will also find that these tools can facilitate a whole new you, and help stabilize a some-times-treacherous emotional journey.

Meditation

Before we start in on a meditation practice, it's important to begin at the bottom. Meditation is not just closing your eyes and letting your mind do the driving. It is a precise, very intentional discipline that will allow you to learn the self-respect necessary for successful weight loss. In order to build a stable meditation practice, we'll start with the 7 Points of Posture. Think of it as a kind of checklist to run through as you settle in to your preferred meditation posture, in order to make sure you are holding yourself with dignity, and not allowing any one part of your body to bear all your weight.

- Begin by going to your chosen meditation spot, if you have already found one. If not, use this time to locate a spot where you will be able to have some privacy every day for at least twenty minutes, and preferably thirty. If you're able to shut the door to make sure you're left alone, so much the better.

• Bring yourself into a cross-legged seated position. If you are prevented from sitting this way for some reason, or suffer from back problems, you may choose to sit in a chair, with your feet flat on the floor.

• The first point of posture is the seat and legs. If you are seated in a cross-legged position, you may want to have a pillow or small cushion under your bottom, to support you. The legs should either have one foot resting in front of the other, or you can bring yourself into full lotus position. If you don't know what that means, don't worry about it. It doesn't affect the experience of meditating. Find a realistic "seat" that you will be able to hold for twenty or so minutes.

• The second point of posture is the eyes, or gaze. Lower your eyelids about halfway, so they are not closed, but not focused on anything. Try to soften your gaze so that it rests about 6-8 feet in front of you, directly over the tip of your nose. This helps you keep from concentrating on anything in the room that may be distracting.

• The third point of posture is the spine, or back, which should be upright, with the bones of the spine stacked one atop the next. However, the posture should not be painful or rigid. Strike a balance between hard and soft. Try to feel your way into the position.

• The fourth point of posture is the shoulders. Hold your shoulders at about the same height, and try to resist scrunching them up near your neck and chin. Try to relax the muscles of the shoulders, and let them be even.

• The fifth point of posture is the neck and throat. The neck should be bent forward slightly, but not excessively, with the chin tucked in slightly. Swallow once, to get rid of any tension in the throat.

• The sixth point of posture is the mouth and tongue. The mouth should be open very slightly, allowing a little space between the upper and lower teeth. This will allow you to breathe through your mouth, if needed, and help keep the jaw relaxed. The tongue should rest on the roof of the mouth, with its tip touching the roof of the mouth.

- The seventh point of posture is the hands. There are many different kinds of hand postures, or *mudras*, in meditation. But for the sake of what we're doing here, we'll just place the hands palms down on the legs, just behind the knees. If your arms are longer, place them over the kneecaps.

- Now that you are settled into your meditation posture, try to find a balance between relaxing into it and slumping over. Slumping is our natural reaction to stress, as it protects the heart and vital organs. But assuming a position of dignity naturally imbues us with the confidence we will need to be in our bodies, and with our bodies, as we strive to find the one that suits us best.

- Begin to notice your breathing. You don't have to do anything. Just notice the feeling of air as it moves in and out of your body, and the way your body moves to accommodate it. As you notice thoughts or storylines in your mind, touch them lightly with your consciousness and say "thinking" to yourself. There is no need to judge the thought, or chase it out of your mind. We're only trying to be with ourselves as authentically as possible. This is what I call the Base Practice. Anytime you want to return to it, please feel free to do so.

- Spend five breaths here, breathing in and out, and labeling your thoughts as they arise. When you feel ready, come out of the meditation.

Follow Up Exercise

This may be the first time you have meditated, so please give yourself a few minutes as you come out of the meditation, so you can readjust yourself to your surroundings. Many times, people are not used to relaxing in this way, so their minds may race around nervously, or even go completely blank. You may have noticed changes in your body as well.

Before you forget, take out your notebook and writing implement, or mini-cassette recorder. Without thinking about it too much, or letting your Internal Editor get the upper hand, write or speak about your experience in the meditation:

- How did it feel to move each part of your body until you found the perfect, balanced meditation posture for you?
- What changes did you notice in your body as you carefully arranged its various parts to find your own 7 Points of Posture?
- How did you feel when you began to notice your breath during the meditation?
- Did you find your mind wandering, or was it pretty calm?
- Did your mind get caught up in any particular storylines? Remember, there is no right or wrong answer. The goal is to be as authentic as possible.
- What changes did you notice in your mind as you kept breathing and labeling your thoughts?
- Finally, what were your overall experiences like during this first meditation?

Once you've written or spoken everything that seems necessary right now, put your notebook or recorder aside. Sit for a moment with your body, allowing whatever feelings you have to just exist. If you hear inner voices of criticism, sit with them. If you hear the sound of your own personal worries, listen to them as well. If you are so inclined, make a note of whatever seems most pressing now. Don't forget to date the page at the top, so you can refer to it at a later date.

Off the Mat Practice

In order to get the full benefit of this program, I ask that you do this meditation once every day for the first week, or longer if you choose, to get familiar with the 7 Points of Posture, and sitting in meditation for twenty minutes or so at a stretch. I know that time is a constant issue in almost everyone's life, so even if you have five minutes at your desk between phone calls, this meditation can help bring greater awareness to your mind-body connection, along with a healthy dose of stress relief as an added bonus.

As well, you can extend this practice a bit more by doing the following once for each day you practice with this chapter: Take one moment—it can literally be a minute, or longer, if you can spare the time—and feel yourself in your body.

"Oh, that's no fun," I can hear you saying. "If I liked doing that, I may not want to/have to lose weight."

Feeling yourself in your body, and making the mental connection that this is what it feels like to be you, right now, begins to establish what so often breaks down for people who carry extra weight—that is, a moment-to-moment awareness of the body. This can also extend to the body's needs, in terms of nutrients, vitamins, sleep, exercise and touch, which become easier and easier to put off if the connection between mind and body is shut off, or you convince yourself that you're not worth nurturing in this way.

All you need to do is stop the racing thoughts of your mind for one instant and say to yourself, "This is what my body feels like, standing still," or, "This is what my body feels like, moving through space." If you have particularly strong feelings come up around this exercise, write about your experiences, or speak about them using your mini-cassette recorder.

If you have a little more time, apply the 7 Points of Posture you found in your meditation to your daily life. As you notice how it feels to be in your body, you may also make a point of noticing how you're holding your hands, or your neck and shoulders. You may become aware of your seat and legs, or how your mouth and tongue feel at this moment. What may seem frivolous to you, or even silly, has a great deal of importance when it comes to losing weight. The connection between the physical functioning of your body and what your mind makes (or doesn't make) of these functions may mean the difference between rooting out an old and unhealthy habit, and keeping things static, exactly where they are now.

Extend Your Practice with Story

A storytelling practice may be new to you. You may not even consider yourself a writer, or have the intention of writing anything more substantial than a birthday card. But you have stories living inside you, and you may not even be aware that you're telling yourself these stories all the time, and making your decisions based on what your mind makes of them.

Your stories may relate to how you look (step in front of a mirror and see if a storyline doesn't immediately get triggered in your mind), how you measure up against others, or even how meetable your future plans and goals may be. Those little voices at the back of your mind, telling you to go towards or away from something, are part of the mechanism inside all of us, that wants to create stories, embellish on the ones we hear, and share them with other people.

All of us have these internal stories running through our minds at all times. Working with our minds in meditation, and then engaging in Follow Up Exercises and Off the Mat Practices will help to get more in touch with how we're using them. But we also have external stories, where we take the raw material of our minds, along with any storylines we're consciously or unconsciously creating, and bring them outside ourselves, by acting on them. We tell tales at gatherings, share petty irritations with mates or friends, or even allow others to create our reality for us, by defining us in a group setting (as "lazy," "friendly," "good-hearted," "someone who eats too much," etc.) The important thing is to become more familiar with the fact that each of us is do-ing this all the time, and then to gain facility with manipulating this process, in order to shift your reality and thereby attain your goals and aspirations.

This week, we'll begin your personal narrative, and add to it over the next eight weeks until you've completely rewritten your internal and external storylines, relative to achieving your weight loss goals. If you haven't written anything before, don't worry about it. We'll move through the process one step at a time, and there will be no tests.

It's best to begin towards the back of your notebook, about thirty or so pages from the end. If you have a notebook with dividers, start at the beginning of the last divider. The front part of your notebook will then become the place you do your weekly exercises and check-ins, and the back will be where you add to your personal narrative over the ensuing weeks. If you prefer, you can begin a computer document for your story, so that you can add to it each week in this way, or even speak your story into your mini-cassette recorder. If you chose this last method, make sure to mark your place with the number counter, or use separate tapes for your exercises and your stories.

To begin, spend a few moments thinking about yourself: where you are in your life physically, mentally, emotionally and spiritually. Then write a paragraph or two explaining who you are and where you find yourself in your life. You may use the third person ("Harry is a thirty-nine year old man who works at a law firm by day and dreams of being a deep-sea fisherman by night.") or the first person ("I am not sure who the real Stella is. Right now, all I know is that she is a nurse, a mother, a sister and a daughter.").

Don't think too much about what you're writing. Often, the first thoughts, images or sentences you have are the best because they're bypassing your Internal Editor. When writers, musicians or even athletes are "on their game," they often seem to achieve their best work while beyond any sort of normal consciousness. Instead, the act of creativity seems to occur most efficiently when it's done outside the reach of our traditional, waking minds.

Things you might address in this paragraph are your age, your family members, your home life, your work life and how you feel about them. You might include some information about your friends and how you spend your leisure time. Finally, you might conclude this section by talking a little about what brought you to this juncture in your life. Have you recently endured a loss? Come to a crossroads? Become sick of the same old, same old? If so, why do you think this has occurred at this time of your life?

When you're finished, read over what you have written, or rewind your tape and listen to what you have recorded. Try to keep voices of criticism from creeping in ("That's not proper grammar," "I hate the sound of my voice," etc.). Instead, just indulge yourself, by listening openly and honestly to what your unconscious mind has brought forth.

In the next chapter, we'll explore what weight is, and what weight stands for in our society. Then we'll begin to look more deeply into how you can get a handle on it in your own life. I've found that each person carries weight differently, and must find a unique path to unlocking the emotional aspects that keep them from shedding it.

What is Weight?

You've completed the first week of your program to achieve your best body, and may be using meditation as a tool for the first time in your life. So far, we've seen that meditation is not just a way to alleviate stress. It can also be very helpful in learning about how our minds and emotions are working with or against the wishes and needs of the body.

This week, we'll start looking into the origins of weight, and how we tend to "use" it in our daily lives. But before we begin, let's take a moment to check in from last week:

- Did you do your daily meditations on the 7 Points of Posture?
- How was your experience of these meditations?
- Did your experience change from day to day, or did it remain relatively constant?
- Were you able to start seeing how your mind is always creating your reality?
- Were you able to record your feelings and experiences after your meditation sessions?
- Did any particularly strong feelings come up for you, and if so, what were they?
- Did you discover anything surprising this week?
- Were you able to do the Off the Mat Practice of noticing yourself in your body at least once per day, even if it was just for a moment?

- If so, how did that feel to you?
- Finally, how are you feeling right now, about yourself, and about your decision to undertake this program?

Please take a moment to record the answers to these questions, as well as any strong feelings you had, using your notebook or mini-cassette recorder. Remember, there is no one in the room with you, and no one will see what you've written. My feelings certainly won't be hurt. So please, be as accurate and authentic as you can. Your duty in performing the meditations and exercises in this program requires you to look within yourself, not within someone else. Necessarily, that means thinking or revealing some unpopular things at times.

When you're finished, take a moment to just sit with yourself as you are now. You may only be a bit closer to your goal of achieving your best body, but I hope you feel as if you're gaining tools to help deal with the stresses inherent in this process.

What Weight Means

The first thing I realized, when confronting my own issues with weight, was that I really had no idea what weight really was, or meant. Sure, I knew that the more pounds you weighed, the higher the number went on the scale, and the larger your clothing had to be. But when I thought about it a little more deeply, I realized that what I thought I knew didn't add up to much at all.

So what exactly is weight?

Webster's Dictionary defines weight as "a measure of the heaviness of an object," or "the force with which a body is attracted to Earth or another celestial body, equal to the product of the object's mass and the acceleration of gravity."

That explains why weight has been synonymous with gravitas, which shares a common root with the word *gravity*, but it doesn't give a three-dimensional portrait of what weight really is, or does, especially on an emotional level.

If we look at synonyms for the word *weight*, we notice that it's often exchanged with units and systems of measure, as well as a measurement of an object's gravitational pull. It's also associated with a counterbalance, as a weight on a balancing scale, or even an object to be lifted so our muscles can develop (this is achieved through isometrics, by pushing or pulling against a certain amount of weight). A weight can hold something else down, or be oppressive in nature. It can also describe a preponderance, or greater part, as well as something important, or with great influence. Finally, the word *weight* is often used to describe classifications in sports such as boxing or wrestling, the thickness of fabrics, and a slant or bias toward or against a person or group.

I can't think of another word in the English language that carries as many conflicting meanings, all in five little letters. If we begin here, we may begin to unravel the confusion that lies at the heart of many weight issues.

Heaviness

When our bodies carry excess weight, we are more attracted to the earth. We exert more force on the ground when we walk or move around. Our center of gravity is often lower. This can mean that we have a chance to become very grounded, or be given a unique opportunity to explore what the earth has to offer.

Earth is one of the four main elements, along with air, water and fire. These elements form the basis for many Asian styles of medicine, which treat spiritual and emotional issues alongside those of the physical body (Chinese medicine adds a fifth element, called *ether*, as does Ayurvedic medicine, while Tibetan medicine adds *Nam-mkha*, or space). All of these elements must be present and balanced for optimum health.

In both medicine and metaphysics, the element of Earth is associated with:

- Growth, and the cultivation of crops
- Stability
- Endurance
- Reliability
- Tranquility
- Solidity
- Duty and groundedness
- Responsibility

- Practicality
- The desire to build and create
- Material comforts
- Caution
- Conservatism
- Sensuality

The quality of heaviness, or attraction to the earth, also has an energetic quality. Usually, it's felt unconsciously, and then acted upon as if it's real. Children, especially, can sense the mood of a room when they walk into it, even if no one says a word. This is how we all pick up on the energy of our exchanges, whether they're with a friend, lover, co-worker or stranger. Earth energy has a strong, solid quality, which may color our exchanges.

If our early lives have been characterized by flightiness (ruled by air), anger (ruled by fire), or intense emotions (ruled by water), perhaps by irresponsible teachers, parents or relatives, we learn to make an internal adjustment. If our mother is light and airy, talking a lot and never listening, we may adopt the state of being physically heavy, in order to balance her need to be light. If our father is rage-filled, directing that energy outward at the rest of the family, a child may learn to become stable and reliable, so as not to incur dad's wrath. Similarly, if we lived with a hyper-dramatic sibling or teacher, we learned to be practical and solid, because there was no room for our emotional lives to develop.

In each of these examples, the person making the adjustment around the other person often creates an internal need to bring them closer to the grounding energy of the earth. As we will see, this often gives rise to an external adjustment as well.

Duty

Many of the people I've worked with, the ones who carry excess weight around with them at least, are often confused about their bodies, and about their own relationship to their bodies. They may be ashamed of their appearance, because it's all too easy for someone else to see that they've eaten too much, or because other people may construe them to be gluttonous, lazy or selfish, when that may be the furthest thing from the truth. Whatever the case, that sense of confusion often prevents them from looking deeper within themselves.

I have found that many heavy people carry weight almost as a sense of duty. In general, abnormal levels of responsibility, anxiety, worry or hardship characterize their lives. One woman, whom I will call Clara, shared her story with me at a storytelling workshop I held in Los Angeles. At six years of age, she cared for three younger siblings while both of her parents worked long hours in a local mine. She was held out of school because the parents did not have any money to pay a babysitter to care for the younger children. This put Clara in charge of cooking for and feeding her brothers and sisters, as well as dressing and bathing them, playing with and entertaining them, and sometimes even teaching them skills, such as ABCs, shoe-tying and even walking.

When Clara told me the story, her eyes filled with tears. The memory of seeing a *Peanuts* cartoon on television, and really wanting to go to school like Charlie Brown and his friends, had stayed with her. Clara's parents came home well after dark, and she told us she could remember feeling the intensity of her fear even today, that someone would break in, or try to hurt her and the other kids. In order to hide her fears from the littler ones, Clara sang to them every night, and urged them to sing along with her. Nursery rhymes, popular songs—it didn't matter. It was the healing power of music that helped Clara survive that time. Her ingrained sense of duty never allowed her to question the needs of her family.

These days, Clara is an extremely responsible woman who works as an emergency room nurse. She says she wants to lose weight and has tried (and stuck to) many diets. But nothing has yielded the results she dreams about so far.

Preponderance

Many others carrying excess weight may want to "throw their weight around," or exert their influence over others. As we saw in Clara's case, duty prevented her from expressing her real feelings—fear of not being up to the task of defending her entire household, and disappointment that she couldn't go to school with the other children of her own age.

Added weight provides a way for many people to achieve the flipside of this. Instead of wanting to engage intimately with others, in the social environment of school for example, heavy people seek to place themselves above it, by accumulating weight and forcing themselves outside the social system.

In many world cultures, excess weight is a sign of prosperity. When times are good, especially after a long period of war or famine, desirable bodies are those with more padding, curves, and greater density. Conversely, when a culture is going through a hard time, or suffering a reversal of fortune, body images seem to adjust, becoming more slimmed-down and body-conscious as food sources dwindle.

Women's fashions are great indicators of the public mood as it relates to weight. For example, during Marie Antoinette's reign, in the 1700s, wealthy members of the royal family (or those that merely wanted to appear that way) made themselves larger by attaching bustles and hooped contraptions to the sides and backs of their skirts, and cinching their waists tight, so they seemed smaller in contrast. Their sleeves were large, their robes long and luxuriously fur-lined, and their wigs piled high with artificial hair like sugary confections. Anything, it seems, to seem bigger and more dominant than the next person.

When the French Revolution restored power to the people, that changed. Sickened by the monarchy's spendthrift ways, the French people insisted on plain clothing that was often handmade, reflecting the common values inherent in the new regime. Because the people viewed themselves as utilitarian, serving the greater good of the nation, their clothing conformed to the body, allowing for the normal motions inherent in many forms of work.

In America, women's fashions were primarily utilitarian during the early part of the twentieth century. Though women with slim hips and cropped hair enjoyed popularity in the 1920s, during the flapper generation, and in the 1960s, emulating the model Twiggy, the preferred body type was curvy and hourglass-shaped, with a 70% hip-to-waist ratio, which suggested the highest fertility rates. In the 1940s, overly thin people were perceived to be nervous and socially maladjusted, even socially withdrawn. Many were given medication or sent to sanatoriums to help them eat and/or sleep, so they could put on more weight.

But as our use of technology increased, following World War II and the Korean War, thin people came to be perceived not only as more desirable, but noble and capable of the sacrifices needed during times of strife. A brief rebellion was waged during the 1960s, when hippies rang in a more tolerant and inclusive view of the human body. But by the 1970s, obsession with self, looks and status converged to create the "Me" Generation.

This fixation on thinness and beauty continued through the 1980s, when the fitness craze was born, and gyms started appearing on every suburban landscape. Thin people were considered appealing and lovable, and many turned to drugs like speed and cocaine to help them stay that way.

Researchers following depictions of models in magazines and on television have found that our bodies are trending more toward thinness each year. As a culture, we are becoming increasingly thin, with hip-to-waist rations that do not suggest childbearing would be welcome, or successful, for that matter.

In an aggressive, self-hating climate like this, who wouldn't want to seem preeminent? Who wouldn't want to reign supreme?

Influence & Importance

Along with the desire to exert one's power or dominance over a situation, a people or a culture, added weight also seems to connote a greater sway or influence. It's hard to imagine Winston Churchill, one of the 20th century's most influential men, without his trademark paunch, or dictator Idi Amin without his imposing girth. Each of these leaders, and many more, almost seem to grow in power as their bodies increase in size.

In keeping with this idea, many people may add excess weight as a way to be seen as influential and valuable to a company, family or relationship. Having the power to produce this effect by indirect means can mean the difference between surviving in a harsh world and not, having the means for continuing and not, and being able to extend your genes, along with your bloodline, into the future.

Additionally, these people may increase their size as a way to become more important to whatever or whomever they treasure. If they feel that they're not being heard, not being appreciated, or don't have the amount of significance for someone else, they may, consciously or unconsciously, allow the extra pounds to slide onto their frames in an effort to be seen, noticed, appreciated or made more significant.

We all want to be important, each in our own way. We want to feel as if we have an impact on the world around us, even if it's just within our own homes. Adding weight is one way to take up more of the room, literally, so you can't be ignored. But ultimately, it may not be the healthiest option to get this important internal need met.

Power

Finally, I have found that weight issues also tend to crop up for people who are interested in, or want to wield power over someone or something. The will to power is as old as humanity itself, but has sometimes endured a bad rap because of its widespread abuse. When most people think of power, they think of Adolph Hitler or other tyrants, or even corporate types taking advantage of people—all relatively negative pictures. But why do we have that vision?

Most of us are taught from an early age not to want power. We're taught to have faith in our families, religions, jobs and relationships, but never to impose our own will or judgements. Power, however, can be a very positive thing. It can help us stick to something, such as a diet or exercise plan. It can help us compel change in a relationship that's not really serving us. It can help motivate complete internal and external transformation, such as when our values are shifting, or our minds are considering another viewpoint. Power over something does not necessarily mean being cruel. Being powerful can also mean becoming a force that puts plans and goals and aspirations into action.

Meditation

This week, we'll start to get more in touch with how the feeling of weight accumulates in our bodies, and also in our minds. Hopefully, you will start to understand some of the unmet emotional needs that may underlie your unconscious desire to carry more weight. Of course, weight issues are not always emotional in nature. Sometimes, a medical issue or simple genetics may be at work. The point is not to make you feel bad about your body, or even wish you had someone else's. It's simply to start looking underneath the surface of added flesh to see if anything needs tending to.

Remember to have your notebook and writing implement handy, or your mini-cassette recorder, if you're working with your experiences in this way.

• Begin by going to your chosen meditation spot and closing the door, if possible. Bring together any materials you may need, such as a pillow, cushion or mat, and arrange yourself into your preferred meditation posture. Make sure to sit upright, in a dignified position, with your legs crossed beneath you for support. If you are seated in a chair, make sure your feet are flat on the floor, and not bent or curled in any way. This will help keep them from falling asleep as well.

• When you feel ready, move through the 7 Points of Posture in your mind, making tiny adjustments as needed. To remind you, the 7 Points of Posture are:

The Seat and Legs: Make sure you're firmly seated in the position of your choice, and have your legs supporting your weight. Let the earth support you completely.

The Eyes and Gaze: Close your eyes halfway, and make your gaze soft, somewhere about 6-8 feet in front of you. Don't focus on any one point in particular.

The Spine: Hold yourself upright, but resist the urge to force your spine into an overly erect posture, or curve it forward to protect your heart. Instead, find a position that stacks up your vertebrae one atop the next.

The Shoulders: Hold your shoulders evenly, without scrunching them up. Try to relax them as you hold them with dignity and intention.

The Neck and Throat: Swallow once, and let your neck and throat be relaxed. Incline the chin slightly, so your gaze is directed slightly downward.

The Mouth and Tongue: Let the tip of the tongue come to rest on the roof of the mouth, and allow the mouth be slightly open, to facilitate breathing.

The Hands: Place the hands palms down on the kneecaps, or just behind the knees on the thighs, depending on how you're put together.

• Once you feel you've achieved the posture you want to keep for the duration of your meditation, begin to notice your breath. It sounds counter-intuitive, but many of us literally don't have the time to notice if we're breathing or not. We leave it up to fate, assuming that our breath will keep coming during every respiration period, as it always has. Right now, just sit with your breath as it moves in and out of your body.

• Allow yourself to feel your body as it sits in meditation. Then, as you begin to notice your thoughts moving through your mind, take a moment to touch them lightly with your consciousness and say "thinking" to yourself. Keep doing this as thoughts or storylines enter your mind.

• People who tend to carry extra weight are often people who have come undone from themselves in some way. They've become distanced from the signals in their own bodies that alert them to mental, physical or emotional trouble. So the next step towards recovering this important link is to reconnect the senses to your meditation.

• Most people find it easiest to do the guided portion of the meditation with eyes closed, so if that works for you, go ahead and close your eyes now. If not, you can also keep your gaze soft and unfocused in front of you, if you like. Bring to mind your eyes, and something you saw today. It could be the grim face of the subway conductor on the way to work, the colorful dresses hanging in the window of a store, or the bowl of ripe strawberries you enjoyed for breakfast. As you picture this image in your mind, notice how it makes your body feel. Do you feel sad for the subway conductor, inspired by the colorful dresses, or hungry at the thought of the strawberries? Whatever the case, notice where those sensations are clustered in your body. Take five breaths in and out here, and then let this image go.

- Now bring your mind to your nose, and something you smelled today. It's not important that it be a "good" thing to visualize. Usually, the first thing that comes to mind is the strongest anyway. So go with the first thing that appears in your consciousness. Try to inhale the smell as if it's there in the room with you right now. Is it the salty smell of the beach? Something flowery, like perfume? Or a proud smell, like the interior of the new car you just bought? Whichever smell you choose, stay with that in your mind for a few minutes, noticing how your emotions are affected by inhaling this smell. Also notice where these feelings seem to occur in your body. For instance, you may find that the beach brings a warm sensation to the back of your shoulders, almost like the sun is hitting them. The flowery perfume may tickle your nose. And the new car smell may make your heart race a little faster, at the idea of taking a drive. Find where the feeling resides in your body. You don't have to do anything about it. Just sit with the image in your mind, and the feeling in your body. Keep breathing.

- Now bring your attention to your mouth and tongue, and something you tasted today. It could be a sweet taste, like a chocolate chip cookie, a savory taste, like the spicy chicken dish you had for lunch, or even a creamy taste, like a fresh fruit smoothie. Whatever made the biggest impression on you in the past 24 hours, bring it to mind now, and try to taste it as if it's in your mouth at this moment. When you're able to visualize this image, try to see how it makes you feel inside. Then try to locate the source of the feeling in your body. Is it in your taste buds? Your stomach? Your heart? Or somewhere else? Hold the image of tasting in your mouth, along with the feeling in your body, as you breathe in and out five times. Notice if your feelings shift at all while you hold this in mind. Then let the image go.

- Now bring to mind your ears, and something you heard today. Again, the first thing that comes to mind is usually the most meaningful for you, even if it's not necessarily the thing you want to remember first. Was the sound you heard short and loud, like a train whistle? Low and soothing, like the comforting voice of your mother? Or staccato, like a musical beat? Hold this image of hearing in your mind, along with any feelings it evokes in you. Take five breaths here, just sitting with your sense of hearing. Then let the image go.

- Finally, bring to mind an image of touching you experienced today. It may have been a soft touch, such as a combed cotton t-shirt, or a rough touch, like the face of an unshaven man. It could even have been a bumpy touch, like the skin of a cucumber. Whatever seems most meaningful for you today, hold that image in your mind. Keep your breathing going at a natural pace. Try to experience this sense as if you're touching the same thing right now. Take five full breaths in and out here, connecting with your sense of touch. Then let the image go.

- Return to your Base Practice, breathing in and out and labeling your thoughts as you notice them in your mind. Touch your thoughts lightly, rather than chasing them out of your mind. You are training yourself to be simultaneously more attuned to the connection between your mind and your body, and less reactive when your mind takes you in a particular direction.

- Come out of the meditation, allowing yourself a few moments to return to normal consciousness.

Follow Up Exercise

After you have given yourself a few moments to re-acclimate yourself to the space around you, take a few moments to record your experiences in the meditation. Many times, my students have not seen the relevance of writing down their experiences while in meditation. But writing these experiences down helps in several ways:

1. First of all, it makes you and your experience more important. Since many people carrying extra weight suffer from a lack of self-esteem, this is an important part of the process.
2. Secondly, it creates a record of what you were going through at a particular point in time. In the future, if you need a map of your progress, you will be able to turn to these pages for support. Since weight loss can be an extended or even lifelong process, this can become all the encouragement you need when you find it hard to go on.
3. Lastly, writing down your experiences has a way of making them more vivid and real to most people. Most of us live our lives in a kind of bubble, where we crave experience and yet are protected from it by emotional and physical buffers we place around ourselves. Having a notebook or mini-cassette recorder to speak into gives you a safe and practical place to begin to remove these buffers from your experience.

So please take few minutes now to write down what you saw, what you heard in your mind, what storylines your mind wanted you to engage in, and how your body was affected by doing this guided meditation. Of course, your writing does not have to be perfect. It doesn't even need to be in whole sentences. Just jotting down a few words, or even a feeling that came up very strongly for you is helpful. And if any memories from your past were activated, make sure to include them as well. All are helpful pieces of the puzzle we're trying to solve in order to facilitate the achievement of your best body.

Off the Mat Practice

Make sure to do this guided meditation on reconnecting with your senses every day of the week you choose to work with this chapter. If you find that it's hard to be consistent, or difficult to find the time, try reminding yourself that it is not selfish to attend to your health. After all, it's your body and mind together that allow you to exist and function in the world. All too often, it's easy to shove that into the background in order to perform our work, take care of others, or reach for goals. But that doesn't help anyone in the long run.

So please find at least twenty minutes each day to devote to your practice. Allow yourself a few moments after each session, in order to record your experiences using your notebook and writing implement or cassette recorder. Remember to date each entry at the top of the page, or with your voice, as you begin recording.

I'd like you to try this Off the Mat Practice as well. Doing it every day of the week will bring you the most benefit, but if you find you only have time to do it once, that's fine.

In this chapter, I talked about what weight means to most people, setting out five major ways that people define weight. Even if this is internalized, and carried around unconsciously, many of us, even if we only have a few pounds to lose, believe certain things about ourselves that can either help us break through the obstacles we set, or keep us cloistered behind them. These often become so deep in us, so entrenched, that they transcend beliefs and become self-definitions. They *are* us, or so we believe:

To remind you of these five major definitions, they are:

1. Heaviness, or Earthiness
2. Duty, or Responsibility
3. Preponderance, or Prosperity
4. Influence & Importance
5. Power

Spend some time just sitting with this list, looking it over to see which one really strikes you as applicable to your own life, or your own circumstances. There may be more than one that applies to you, but for now, just choose the one that seems *really* like you.

When you have chosen the definition you most want to work with, open your notebook and find a fresh page. Date the entry at the top. Then, off the top of your head, write or speak about the things that immediately come to mind when you think of that word, or that way of defining weight. Does a particular face come to mind, or a friend, mate or relative? Do certain words, of criticism perhaps, come to mind? Do you immediately start to relive a certain event from your life, or a fantasy projection into the future?

Just record anything that comes to mind now, making a promise to yourself to be as open and honest as you can with what you experience. You are not here to please anyone; that doesn't do anyone any good. If any mental connections occur to you, make sure to write them down, for further exploration in the future. An example would be the mental connection between power, say, and your early relationship with your father, which made you want to eat more than necessary. You will no doubt have your own connections that mean something for your life.

When you have identified the weight-defining word or phrase that best describes your situation, and done your free writing around this topic, sit for a few minutes with your feelings. Notice how it feels to be in your body. Try to contact each individual part of your frame at least once per day, even if that means that you are only doing a quick scan.

Then, try to extend your practice by becoming more aware of how you act out this weight-defining word or phrase in your everyday life. If your chosen word or phrase is "Duty, or Responsibility," try to notice when you accept more work than you want to accept at your job, hoping that it will endear you to your boss or co-workers. You might notice that you feel more exhausted than usual after work. Or you may notice that a friend's problems almost become *your* problems, because of the way you've become so involved in her life.

At least once per day, notice one way in which you are physically enacting this weight-defining word or phrase. It may be very hard to do at first, because most of us are not used to noticing our moment-to-moment behavior, feelings, or both together. But with practice, I'm sure you can become more aware of how you're behaving, and most importantly, how you're feeling when you behave this way.

Once you notice that you're acting out of this particular place, just relax into it. You don't have to chastise yourself for being too dutiful, or vow to make behavioral adjustments. For now, it's great to see how you may be inadvertently allowing a common definition for weight to reside in your subconscious mind. Noticing this doesn't make you stupid, it makes you courageous enough to take action.

Immediately following these times when you notice yourself behaving out of this place, take a few minutes to write (or speak into your mini-cassette recorder) about your experience. Make sure to include a description of the situation as it unfolded, your emotions relative to the situation and then, if possible, where those feelings were located in your body. Did you feel a knot growing in your stomach? A pounding headache, right between your eyes? Or something else entirely?

Over the next few weeks, we'll develop strategies for deepening this sense of awareness, and come up with suggestions on how to wean yourself away from potentially self-destructive behaviors. Know that if any truly painful feelings come up for you, you can always sit in meditation, using the guided prompts I've supplied, or in your Base Practice, by labeling your thoughts and watching your breath. Even if you're upset, your breathing will slow, your heart rate will come down, and you'll enjoy a renewed sense of your own purpose.

Extend Your Practice with Story

Last week, you began to tell your story, beginning with a paragraph or two about yourself and your life as it is now. You may have written or spoken about your job, your family, your downtime or added other details. Did it feel safe to reveal yourself in this way?

Now that a week has passed, read over what you wrote last week. Do you still feel the same way about your life? It's not important to go back and change the writing you did. Instead, just look at where you were a week ago compared with where you are now. Many things may contribute to a shift in perspective, including your meditation sessions.

Then, continue your story by writing another paragraph or two about your body. Remember, it doesn't have to be perfectly spelled; it doesn't have to be correct grammatically. It merely has to reflect what you truly feel about yourself, in an authentic way.

Try to describe your body. What shape does it have? Are any features similar to those of your other family members? What does your body have that you especially like? What does your body have that you especially dislike? What functions does your body perform for you that you're grateful to have?

Then describe what it feels like when your body is still. Can you compare it with something else you've seen, such as a flower, a comfortable chair, or an animal? What are the feelings that come up for you when you fully inhabit your body? Do you want to run, or are you enticed to stay awhile?

Finally, describe what it feels like when your body is moving through space. Are you aware of each moment your feet contact the ground? Do you feel like you're floating, or completely earthbound? What are the emotions that come up for you as you experience your body moving through space?

If you feel inspired to write or record more than a paragraph or two, please feel free to continue. Sometimes, the act of spilling out our thoughts, especially while they're fresh in our minds, can be therapeutic. But since most everyone has time constraints of one type or another, just writing a few paragraphs is great, too. Remember to read over what you've written before putting it aside for this week.

Next week, we'll begin to discuss how weight is "lost," and how the process of losing weight can often bring up unexpected personal issues. Until then, enjoy practicing with your own definition of weight. Know that you are moving closer to your best body every single day.

"Losing" Weight

In the second week of our program, we'll take what we learned last week and integrate it with your experiences in your individual meditations and Off the Mat Practice sessions. In doing this, we'll begin to see how the act of feeling yourself in your body, and reaching towards your weight loss goals affects your emotions, and how it may continue to affect you long after you stop dieting.

Becoming more aware of the ever-present interactions between your emotions and body may protect you from unconscious eating, but it may also become the foundation of your awareness, which can be used to protect you from many related issues unique to the weight loss process.

But first, let's take a moment to check in from last week:

- Did you have a chance to do your meditation exercises every day of the week?
- If not, what kept you from meditating every day?
- What strategies might you adopt to help yourself stay on track?
- Were your sessions usually about 20-30 minutes in duration? Longer? Shorter?
- Did you spend a few minutes writing down or speaking about your experiences in the meditations?
- If so, did you notice one particular experience you kept having?

- If so, how did that experience make you feel?
- Where was the feeling located in your body?
- If you didn't have one overriding emotion in your meditation sessions, did your emotions fall into a particular category, or were they all over the map?
- How did it feel to start feeling your mind and body operating together in this way?
- Did you notice any old memories or storylines coming up for you?
- If so, what were they?
- Were you able to engage in the Off the Mat Practice on defining the meaning of weight in your life?
- Which meaning did you choose to work with?
- What made this definition the most potent for you at this time?
- When you noticed yourself acting out of this place in your daily life, what kinds of feelings were evoked?
- Where was this feeling located in your body?
- Was the feeling located in one area, or more than one area?
- Did you find yourself chastising yourself for acting out of this place?
- If so, were you able to relax into just noticing the behavior each day?
- Did you spend some time writing or speaking about the experiences you had in your Off the Mat Practice?
- Lastly, did you notice that your awareness of your thoughts, feelings and bodily sensations were increased during the week?

Once you have spent some time writing or speaking your answers to these questions, spend a few minutes just checking in with where you are right now. Notice any thoughts that don't seem to want to leave your mind, or any scenarios that are still playing out from your day. Take note of any strong emotions as well as any strong physical sensations, without trying to chase them out. Just notice where you are in all areas of your life now. Let everything co-exist together. Where you are is exactly where you need to be at this moment.

The Three Poisons

We're all familiar with poisons. They come in bottles with skulls and crossbones on them, warning us what might happen if we take them

into our bodies. Instead of assisting our systems in their daily functioning, they hinder and sometimes stop them altogether. Most of us avoid
poisons, simply because they're harmful.

Buddhists believe that there are three major causes of *dukkha*, or suffering. Suffering does not have to mean intense pain, or constant reminders
of failure. In this instance, it's subtler than that. What it means, in essence,
is to be trapped in a cyclical world of one's own creating. Weight, and the
act of losing weight, can seem very much like that.

The three poisons are passion, aggression and ignorance, and are
depicted as a rooster, snake and pig at the center of many Tibetan
thangkas, or religious paintings. These poisons are said to prevent
us from being truly enlightened, which I take to mean both spiritually and physically. Each poison has a very important connection
to carrying and losing weight, and to the foundation within each
of us that many inadvertently contribute to our keeping unwanted
weight on.

Passion, or Desire

In our culture, passion is used interchangeably with the strong will
to do something. We use it in a complimentary way, to indicate that
someone cares very much about what she's doing, or has a burning need
to solve a problem, or utilize an inborn skill.

But if we look under the surface of the word, passion is another
way of desiring something or someone. Perhaps we look at a model's
body and desire it so much, we're willing to starve ourselves to have
it. Maybe we like someone so much we're willing to deny ourselves
adequate nutrition so the person will like us.

In this instance, passion is also synonymous with greed or lust. We
may become greedy about food, hoarding it for ourselves. We may never
be satisfied with what we have, or be worried that it will somehow be
taken from us. One friend I have sheepishly admits to loving a certain
kind of chocolate sold only in England. Though there are a few specialty
stores which sell this chocolate, or can order it for her, she prefers to
keep at least a box of chocolate bars in reserve, hidden in her cupboard.
This is passion at its most heightened, and shows how it can color our
behaviors in strange and not-so-strange ways.

People struggling with weight, mentally, emotionally and/or physically, often have trouble with the concept of passion. After all, we've been taught that intrepid explorers founded our country by forging new paths over treacherous mountain paths. Desire had to play some part in that. And of course, passion for helping people, through science or an artistic pursuit, can end up greatly benefiting a culture. But understanding how the poison of passion helps us to stay enslaved to weight requires some additional internal work.

Perhaps it's easiest to start with our own concepts of our bodies. If we try to visualize ourselves in our mind's eye, it's not too difficult, because we have the aid of mirrors, and can see ourselves all the time, if we choose. Of course, we know that our bodies continue to age, and that this process will bring physical decline. But on some level, we also believe, as we live our day-to-day lives, that our bodies are permanent. What we see in the mirror is real, and our minds immediately do two things: try to cement this moment so that our sense of self is bolstered, and form an opinion about what we see. Passion is an integral part of both.

Because seeing and imagining our bodies is such a loaded issue, carrying with it the seeds of our biological survival as well as our ability to form relationships, mate and perpetuate our species, it is one of the main areas we use to form our sense of self. Our skin provides the boundaries of our physical existence. Our DNA determines how we will be formed, or which diseases might attack our cells with greater ease. The way our brains store and retrieve information helps or hinders us from what we want to attain. All of that combines into the way we perceive ourselves, or our sense of self. We don't even have to think about it; we just know.

Passion comes in when we feel that sense of self being threatened. It is the fuel for our fire, that spark that has us reacting to a situation before we've had even a second to determine what the best course of action may be. It's the impatient urge to buy that untested diet pill or to stop eating altogether, so we can reach that all-important goal sooner. It's the push to eat more than we need, and the inexorable pull to protect what we have, because losing it would be intolerable.

In short, passion is the poison that keeps us obsessing about food, the way we look, and the way we want to look, sometimes simultaneously.

Aggression, or Anger

The sense of self is also important to understanding the concept of aggression or anger. Maybe we believe we understand anger. Someone irritates us, and we blow up. We hear about a perceived injustice, and we get riled up so we can change it. Our boss tries to claim credit for our work, and we burn inside, just itching to react in some way.

But this is a simplistic understanding of this very complicated emotion. In short, aggression and anger arise when what we believe to be true, or want to be true, is thwarted in some way. We perceive that our desires have been rejected by some cosmic power, and our reaction is called anger. Related emotions include hatred, jealousy and cruelty, among others.

Anger stems from our sense of self, or at least the part of it that believes that it is the *only* self, or the *most important* self. This self is an illusion, and when it believes it has lost control over something it believes to be important, it produces an equally illusory emotion, anger. Whatever is causing us pain has got to stop, and we react quickly and decisively, in order to stop the pain from hurting us any further.

In this heightened state of emotion, anger's heated energy is moving through us, but we seldom have the equanimity to stop ourselves from reacting in a negative way. Instead, this illusionary sense of self, along with the reactive emotions it produces, leaves us open to internal and external dangers.

Anger begins in the amygdala, the part of our brains that help us identify and react to perceived threats. This often provokes a reaction before the cortex, or reasoning center, can determine the best course of action relative to this threat. Thus, our survival instinct supercedes our ability to logically weigh the consequences of our actions.

At the same time, our muscles tense, and the brain releases catecholamines, or neurotransmitters, which provide energy and heat to the body. Respiration and blood pressure rise. Our "color" also rises, as blood is pumped into our face and extremities. Adrenaline and noradrenaline are also released, keeping the body's chemistry in a vigilant, alert-ready state.

But the internal effects of anger do not stop there. Once we no longer perceive a particular threat, the body begins to relax, but very slowly.

The "rush" that comes from adrenaline in the bloodstream can last for many hours, or even days. This can often leave us open to experiencing anger again, even if the irritation is smaller and less significant.

Externalizing anger rarely makes it better. As we experience these disturbing inner changes, we may feel pushed to relieve the tension. We may yell, gesture broadly or condemn the source of our irritation. We may become overly critical, experience resentment or bitterness, or even lose sleep over our anger. Lastly, we may turn the anger we feel back on ourselves, in the form of envy, depression or apathy. But even though "unloading" our anger, on ourselves or others, may help us feel better temporarily, the original source is still there, and may even continue to provoke us before our bodies can ratchet down from our adrenaline "high." Either way, our bodies continue to experience anger in the same way.

People carrying extra weight often have ambivalence about aggression or anger. Some find it hard to express anger, and instead harbor it inside. Others may feel unable to hold all their anger, and feel the need to behave aggressively towards others. What most can agree on is that understanding anger is crucial to understanding weight. Unexpressed or misunderstood anger can cause us to feel badly about our bodies, or can even manifest in aggressive behavior towards ourselves, such as crash diets or invasive surgery.

Anger is a strong emotion that is also measured according to societal rules. In many families or other group situations, it is established early on that one person has the right to express his or her anger freely, while others are prevented from expressing theirs. In some cultures, expressing anger is so difficult or unacceptable that people are willing to kill themselves, with suicide or a manifested problem like heart disease or cancer, rather than break the taboo. But anger is energy first and foremost. And because of this, it can also be transformed, with effort and training, into an emotion no more harmful than breathing in and breathing out.

Ignorance

Sometimes called delusion, ignorance is the state of perceiving the world as something other than what it truly is. We believe what we see, or what we're told, or the "common wisdom" of a situation. Instead of using our senses to perceive what is, we buy into what others believe. We allow them to tell us how things are, or even how we should feel about our bodies. This can color how we act towards ourselves, or how we decide to treat others.

It's no accident that ignorance is portrayed as a pig in traditional Tibetan paintings. Pigs symbolize laziness, since they rarely leave their mud wallows, other than to eat and drink. Many religions, including Judaism and Islam, forbid the eating of pork because of the pig's unclean, omnivorous diet. One common belief is that pigs will literally eat anything put in front of them, including feces.

The act of carrying extra weight is also associated with some of these same qualities. As a society, we equate heaviness with laziness, or call heavy people "pigs." We assume that heavy people wallow around in a world of their own creation, and that they can't or won't do anything to get out of it. Many believe that heavy people are unclean, and that they, too, would eat anything put in front of them.

As such we may, intentionally or unintentionally, associate the quality of heaviness with ignorance, or lack of wisdom. If they only knew better, we think, they wouldn't carry so much weight. Why don't they eat more fruits and vegetables, instead of pigging out at fast food restaurants all the time? *Don't they know? Can't they understand?*

Some people who carry extra weight may indeed not know about healthier dietary choices. But ignorance about healthy choices can cut both ways. A person who believes that a "normal" American diet of hamburgers, pizza, french fries and sugary sodas is somehow healthy may find benefit in learning about how to make food choices that can help them lose weight, lower their cholesterol, or avoid diabetes. But a person who projects all of his or her unexamined issues onto others (heavy people are a popular target) may find that examining his or her own ignorance to be just as helpful.

Of course it's important to understand how carrying too much weight is detrimental, and even outright dangerous, to overall health. But if we don't want to fall to the poison of ignorance, we must dedicate ourselves to digging deeper, to *not* taking things at face value. Instead, we're urged to look at both sides of the coin.

In Chinese astrology, the Year of the Pig heralds goodwill and prosperity. In these times, there is generally plenty for all, and sensual pleasures take precedence. Though most people usually find themselves focusing on security, it's easy to fall into excessive behaviors in eating, drinking, gambling or sex. People born during the Year of the Pig are said to have steady, faithful personalities, characterized by friendliness and generosity. Sometimes, Pigs can be blunt in speech and actions, but find it very hard to refuse a request. This can leave them indecisive, or at the mercy of other, stronger personalities. Still, the Year of the Pig is a popular year for Chinese parents to try and have a child.

According to The Humane Society, many myths about pigs are also untrue:

- Though we use the phrase "sweat like a pig" frequently, pigs do not sweat. Mud cools them off, and this has led, perhaps unfairly, to their being labeled unclean.
- Pigs are very hygienic animals that will not live or eat around waste.
- According to Pennsylvania State University professor Stanley Curtis, pigs can respond to verbal cues and even play computer games, using their snouts. When trying to hit a particular target, his research pigs scored over 80%.
- Pigs can learn their names within 2-3 weeks, and often respond when called.
- Pigs have a sense of direction, and many can find their way home, if lost.
- Pigs are social animals that communicate with gestures of friendship and grooming. They sleep together, and form stable social groupings, according to dominant behaviors.
- Pigs also locate food using social means, by watching each other and following the pig that finds food.
- Pigs have a complex language of sounds to communicate the best times to mate, to suckle, or to indicate distress.

The point is that, despite the conventional wisdom, we don't know all there is to know about pigs, just as we don't know everything about the human body, its unique nutritional needs, or the myriad of reasons it accumulates and stores extra weight. The best approach to ignorance is to remain as open as possible, despite our desire to know all there is to know.

Ignorance, like passion and anger, can be transformed into a helpful emotion, capable of fostering curiosity, sparking debate or asking questions, rather than shutting down, tuning out, or making up your mind beforehand.

Transforming Difficult Emotions

Meditation is one very important tool to help transform passion, aggression and ignorance, as well as the behaviors they evoke in us, into something more positive, or at least healthier for our long-term development. Though meditation doesn't magically "heal" these emotions, or force them out of your life, it will, over time, give you the space you need to see the issue clearly, and to not fall immediately into a reactive way of behaving.

How it works is this: when someone or something "triggers" us, we usually respond by forming a mental opinion about this person or event, and then having an emotional response. In a certain way, this is hard-wired into us. It may happen when someone overlooks us, insults us, or assaults us verbally or physically. It may happen when someone loves us, but not in the way we want. It may happen when we get the job of our dreams, but then have to make a series of uncomfortable changes.

So the point is not to rid ourselves of this reactivity. I like to think that it may be possible, but I haven't met a human being yet who doesn't have it happen from time to time. Reactivity can help us to swerve our car into an empty lane when someone cuts into ours without looking. It can help us realize something is wrong in our bodies when we aren't breathing "right." And it can even help us leave behind a bad situation for one that may assist our development in the long run.

But too much reactivity means that we're not living consciously. In a sense, we're becoming enslaved to the people and events around us, always reacting to whatever happens, and never acting in a way that empowers us. If you've decided to undertake a new way of looking at food and eating, or even incorporating some exercise into your schedule, you've already taken one step towards being more conscious. You've recognized an issue in your life, identified one possible solution, and taken action towards meeting your goal (At least you've gotten this far in the book!). Now, it's time to work on keeping our minds open, but most importantly, aware on a moment-to-moment basis.

"Losing" weight is often thought of as a brief program of semi-starvation followed by the buying of new clothes, the fielding of compliments, and maybe getting a new romantic partner. While we diet, we dream about all the foods we will eat when we've arrived at our goal. But of course, that thinking only leads to disappointment. As soon as we've reached our weight loss goal, we eat all the same old foods again, as if the preceding three or six or nine months were some sort of exercise in self-denial. Inevitably, the pounds start to creep back on, and we're in the bookstore again, looking for the next big diet that will "cure" our problem with extra weight. Transforming negative emotions may be very applicable in a situation like this. If we're fired up to lose weight, we may be acting out of passion. If we undertake a diet that leaves us hungry and needing more nutrients, perhaps we're acting out of aggression. And if we believe that somehow dieting today will mean not having to diet tomorrow, then we may be acting out of ignorance.

Achieving our best body, the one that perfectly right for us, means that we must understand our emotions before we begin to transform them. We must understand that our actions, as well as our thoughts, can undermine or completely derail us before we've reached our goals. And we must make a commitment to being in our bodies *all the time*, so we can begin to sort out the tangled nest of emotions, thoughts and physical sensations that characterize all human beings.

Once you are able to obtain a level of moment-to-moment awareness like this, you can use the meditations and exercises in this book to help you make better choices for yourself as you achieve your best body. With that in mind, let's get started on this week's meditation. We will discover more about transforming negative emotions in the next chapter.

Meditation

This week, we'll delve a little deeper into the three poisons, and find out how they may be enacting themselves in your life and your stories, perhaps without your knowledge. You do not have to be a Buddhist, nor do you have to follow any religion, really, to work with the three poisons. The reason I find them helpful in a weight loss program is because they start to help us see how we're not seeing ourselves. This may include inflated or under-developed senses of self, or just how we begin to touch our stories, so they effect not just the times we get together with our families to reminisce, but in every moment of every day.

During this meditation, try to pay special attention to how your feelings come up, as well as locating where these feelings may be strongest in your body. This will help provide clues as to the type of inner work you may need to do in tandem with any diet or exercise plans you may have.

- Begin in a seated position, with your legs crossed, or seated in a chair, with your feet flat on the floor. For this meditation, try to wear light clothing, if it's not too cold where you live, and leave your feet bare. We're trying to get you in touch, as much as possible, with the feeling of being supported by the earth. Wearing lighter clothing and foregoing shoes will also help you become more aware of your body, and how feelings lodge themselves in its tissues.

- Bring yourself into your preferred meditation posture, remembering the 7 Points of Posture.

- First, bring your awareness to your legs and seat. Provide a comfortable yet stable foundation for your practice, by finding the right balance of body over legs. Feel the earth under your legs and/or feet, providing the support you need.

- Now bring your attention to your eyes and gaze, directing the eyes slightly downward, tilting the chin, and softening the gaze.

- Now bring your attention to your spine. Hold yourself upright and dignified, without tightening your muscles too much.

- Next, focus on your shoulders. Make them the same height, and try to let the muscles relax as you find the right pose for you.

- Bring your attention to your neck and throat. Swallow once, and relax the neck as you direct your gaze downward.

- Next, bring your attention to your mouth and throat. Rest the tongue lightly on the roof of the mouth. Let your mouth be open slightly.

- Finally, bring your attention to your hands, by resting them lightly just behind the knees, or draped over the kneecaps, if your legs are longer.

- Take five full breaths here, relaxing into your meditation posture. Just notice the breath as it moves in and out of your body, without trying to do anything about it.

- When you feel ready, begin to connect each of your senses to your meditation. Start with your fingers, and notice how the air moving past them affects the sensitive nerve endings there. Then notice any sounds, however slight, in the room with you. Next, bring your attention to your eyes, and just notice whatever is in your field of vision, without moving your gaze in any way. Swallow once, and see if there are any lingering tastes in your mouth. Lastly, inhale deeply, and notice any smells in the atmosphere around your body.

- Take five full breaths here, experiencing all your senses as they work together to bring you sensory information, and filter it so you can interpret it.

- Now bring to mind a recent event in which you felt really passionate. It could be passionate love, as with a child, or passionate hatred of your own body. Just think about this instance for a few breaths, trying to visualize it as best you can. Notice where the feelings are located in your body, such as a surging heart, faster breath, or an aching stomach. Sit with those feelings for a few breaths, and then let them go.

- Let the image go as well, and begin your Base Practice. When you notice a thought in your mind, or a storyline taking you away from the present moment, say "thinking" to yourself.

- Now bring to mind a recent event in which you felt aggressive. This may be a competitive sport, a meeting at work, or something you directed at an unsafe motorist on the freeway. Just imagine that moment in your mind as you take your next few breaths. Notice where the feelings associated with this moment are lodged in your body. Are they in your shoulders? Your eyes? Your ankles? Then let the image go.

- Return to your Base Practice for a few breaths, labeling your thoughts and returning to the breath.

- Now bring to mind an instance when you felt ignorant, or came into contact with ignorance. This may have been yourself, as you learned something you hadn't previously known, or when someone you interacted with displayed something they didn't know. What are the feelings that come up for you when you remember this interaction? Where do these feelings manifest themselves in your body? Sit with these emotional and physical feelings for a few breaths, and then let the image go.

- Return to your Base Practice for five breaths, labeling your thoughts as they arise, and letting them leave you on your out breath. Come out of the meditation.

Follow Up Exercise

Allow yourself a few minutes to come back into your regular consciousness. Then, using your notebook and writing implement or mini-cassette recorder, record the experience you had during your meditation session:

- Did you remember the 7 Points of Posture?
- Were you able to find your way into your meditation posture pretty easily?
- Were you able to connect each of your senses to your meditation without difficulty?
- Did any feelings come up for you when you were connecting your five senses?

- If so, where were they centralized in your body?
- Was there a common place, or did your feelings seem to move around?
- When you visualized a recent event involving passion, what person or event did you see in your mind's eye?
- How did seeing this image make you feel?
- When you visualized a recent event involving aggression or anger, what person or event did you see in your mind's eye?
- How did seeing this image make you feel?
- When you visualized a recent event involving ignorance, what person or event did you see in your mind's eye?
- How did seeing this image make you feel?
- Did you have any memories come up during your meditation?
- Finally, are there any feelings left over from your meditation session? If so, note them down, without feeling the need to judge or analyze them.

Make sure to record all the experiences you had during your meditation session immediately afterwards, so you don't forget anything. Many ideas, images, feelings or memories can come up while meditating, because the brain is particularly open to receiving (or retrieving) this information. Even if you saw, heard, smelled, tasted or touched something inside that isn't on this list, include it in your record.

Also, make sure to record any memories that came to mind while you were mediating. I have had people make connections between passion, Martha Graham and being embarrassed about going to the ballet with their mothers, for instance, or ignorance, eating pork, and their brother's six months as a vegetarian. Even if it seems insignificant to you now, please take the time to record it. In time, it may make more sense, or be able to be woven together with other experiences to form a complete picture.

Off the Mat Practice

During the week (or more) you decide to practice with "losing" weight and the three poisons, make sure to leave at least twenty to thirty minutes each day to do your meditation practice. This is a way of engaging with yourself daily, and checking in with your mind, body and emotions simultaneously, without resorting to self-involved or inappropriate behavior.

As well, try to keep reminding yourself to be present in your body when you can, even if it's literally for sixty seconds each day. Feel yourself as you sit still, as you move through space, and as your internal life, of thoughts and feelings, interacts with your external self, and the individual parts of your body.

Then, in order to extend your practice into your daily life, try this exercise:

On the first day of the week, go to a fresh page in your notebook and date the entry at the top. Then write (or speak into your recorder) the word *Passion*. Draw a line under the word. Underneath, without thinking about it too much, write down all the words, phrases, feelings or images you associate with that word. It could be a person, a place, a memory—anything goes, so let your imagination run wild. Take about 2-5 minutes to do this, no longer. Otherwise, the part of the mind that wants to judge or analyze becomes dominant.

Then, write the word *Aggression*, and draw a line under it. List all of the words, phrases, associations, images, people, places and things that come to mind when you see or hear that word. Does it affect any part of your body in particular? Does it bring up any memories, or cause you to think about the future? Again, don't over-think it. Just let your most imaginative mind take over for about 2-5 minutes, sketching out a verbal picture of what this word means to you.

Then do the same for the word *Ignorance*. Write the word down, underline it, and begin to list all the associations you have with that word, whether they're visual, auditory, olfactory, tactile or gustatory in nature. Now that you have had a few weeks of practicing with your mind, you may notice that your creativity comes forward more easily, and with a lot less judgment attached to it. Let yourself be the wild, creative person you are inside. That person has a lot of wisdom to share.

Then, on the second day of the week, go to a fresh page in your notebook, and date the entry at the top. If you are speaking into a tape recorder, you can do this with your voice as well. Write the word *rooster*, and then draw a line under it. Underneath that, begin to write down or speak all of the things you associate with this word. It could be an image, a person, a style of dress—whatever comes to mind is valuable, so write it down! Spend about 2-5 minutes here, just scribbling all you see in your mind's eye that relates to the word.

Then, write the word *snake*, and underline it in your notebook. Without allowing your rational mind to creep in too much, write down, as fast as you can, all the people, places, things, feelings, and memories you may have with the word *snake*. Don't be afraid to let the ugly parts of yourself show, because no one is watching.

Then do the same for the word *pig*. Write down the first things that come into your mind, because those are usually the richest and most meaningful for you. Spend about 2-5 minutes writing down everything you see, hear, smell, touch or taste when you think of this word. Then try to locate any feelings you have about it, and where they're residing in your body. Put your notebook aside, and spend the rest of the week letting it all sink in.

Extend Your Practice with Story

Last week, you added a few more paragraphs to your story as it relates to achieving your best body. So far, you have taken the time to describe yourself and your life, as well as the way you see yourself. You may have even become more in touch with the way you feel when you're fully inside your body, emotionally present and aware.

Next week, we'll continue building your story, to include how you would prefer to feel about your body. Most of us, when asked this question, may want to rattle off, without thinking, "Oh, I'd prefer to have Kate Moss' body," or "'I want to be able to eat anything I want, and never gain an ounce." But to be so flip about our bodies, which house our souls, provide us with support, and facilitate all of our movements, is to overlook and devalue ourselves. And if we devalue ourselves, chances are, we will allow others to do the same.

Go back to your notebook, and find the place you left off in your story last week. If you're using a cassette recorder, change tapes, if necessary, or locate the place you left off last week. Then read over or listen to what you wrote last week. Resist the impulse to go back and change what you said, or to embellish what you wrote. These words were true for you then, and it's important to allow them to stand on their own.

Then spend some time thinking about how you would prefer your body to be. Start from the inside, describing how you would like to feel in your body, both when it's still and then when it's moving through space. Use visual words and comparisons to various objects to illustrate how your feelings resonate inside you, and to give them more texture.

Then move outward. Describe how you would like your body to look, staying away from specifics such as wearing a particular size or weighing a certain number of pounds. Instead, talk about how the shape or size of your body might be shifted to align with what your mind imagines for it. Talk about how your feelings about your body might change if these external changes were to occur. And finally, describe how other people might perceive you once your body has changed in this way.

Take all the time you need to write a paragraph or two on how you would prefer to think and feel about your body, and how you perceive your body changing to come into greater alignment with whatever your mind sees. Remember to let yourself be authentic and free as you perform this exercise, reporting honestly on what you perceive right now to be true. If your Internal Editor shows up for a visit, insist that he or she wait outside until you're finished. As always, if you have the time, energy or inclination to write or speak longer, that's great. If not, no worries. You'll derive the same benefits either way.

Before setting your work aside for the week, read over what you have written, or rewind your tape and listen to what you have recorded. Make sure to stay vigilant, as if listening to a valued friend. You are learning to trust *your* experience as much as that of someone else. Hear what you appear to be saying on the surface, as well as what you may be yearning for underneath your words. This will become easier as the next few weeks pass.

Next week, we'll look into the issue of taste, which can be a loaded one for people carrying added weight. For now, though, know that your meditation practice is helping you become more familiar with yourself, and therefore, to know what your body needs and doesn't need to keep it functioning at its healthiest level.

Chapter Four

> "Nothing takes the taste out of peanut butter quite like unrequited love."
>
> -- Charles M. Schulz, from *Peanuts*

A Matter of Taste

It has been said that eating too much, and adding extra weight to one's body, is a cry for help. It has also been said that extra weight symbolizes pounds of pain, and that to lose them is to rid oneself of that pain forever. Eating too much has been equated with trying to recapture the sense of being loved. And finally, it has been suggested that fat is a feminist issue, and that carrying extra weight wouldn't be shameful if our systems weren't patriarchal in nature. All of these are probably true, on some level.

But this week, we'll delve into an issue that most people who want to lose weight can identify with: taste. We all have unique ways of eating, savoring and enjoying food. Some people even go so far as to adopt an eating style, and form a real relationship with food, as they would with a living person. We'll explore a new way to look at this particular sense, and try to identify ways you may be using stories to help or hinder your own weight loss goals.

But first, let's take a minute to check in from last week:

- Did you get to do your meditation exercises every day of the week?
- If so, what were your overall experiences like during your meditation sessions?
- Did you have any persistent feelings that came up for you when you imagined a recent event in which you experienced passion?

67

- If so, what were they, and where were they located in your body?
- Did you have any persistent feelings that came up for you when you imagined a recent event in which you experienced aggression?
- If so, what were they, and where were they located in your body?
- Did you have any persistent feelings that came up for you when you imagined a recent event in which you experienced ignorance?
- If so, what were they, and where were they located in your body?
- Did you spend some time after each meditation session, recording your experiences?
- Were you able to do the Off the Mat Practice, free-associating on passion, aggression and ignorance?
- If so, how did that make you feel?
- Did any images, feelings of memories come up repeatedly as you did this exercise?
- Were you able to do the Off the Mat Practice, free-associating on the words *rooster*, *snake* and *pig*?
- If so, what were your experiences like?
- Did you have any particular feeling come up more than once? If so, what was it?
- Finally, did you feel drawn towards any one of these in particular? If so, which one?

Spend a few moments writing or speaking your answers to these questions. Then, just sit with your feelings right now. How do you feel? How does your body feel? Have you noticed any changes since we began this program?

Write or speak about your experience right now, here, today. All of it has value.

Learning to Taste

Taste may be the most sensual of all the senses. It involves taking something into your mouth, a gesture that leaves us vulnerable and open, quite literally. Because of that, the sense of taste involves trust. Usually, it takes us a good deal of time, perhaps years, before we would be able to trust a person to stick his or her fingers into our mouths. But for some reason, we give this power to food far more readily.

We owe our sense of taste largely to our ability to smell. Scientists estimate that 80-90% of what we perceive as taste is linked to our olfactory system. When our nasal passages are stuffed up, food tastes different. When we have a head cold, we may be unable to taste at all. So it is our ability to smell food and other stimuli that enables us to taste.

Secondarily, it is our ability to respond to tastants, or dissolved molecules and ions, which allow us to experience the sense of taste. Each of us has multiple taste receptor cells, clustered together in the taste buds on our tongues. A pore in each taste bud allows the food we eat to interact with these tastants.

There are five main types of taste: salty, sour, sweet, bitter and umami (a response to glutamates, like those found in processed foods, also called savory). Each has its own unique way of admitting (salty and sour) and binding to (sweet, bitter and umami) ions of each taste type. When this has been done successfully, a message will be carried back to the brain through an ATP-releasing synapse.

This message first gets processed in the brain stem, or medulla oblongata, which regulates respiration, blood pressure and heart rate, among other functions. It is then passed to the forebrain, where our sense of reasoning lies. Here, we decide if a taste is "good" or "bad," "appealing" or "unappealing." It also starts to explain why, as humans, we seem to have to make these emotional connections with the food we eat, or the various events in our lives.

Anyone who's ever struggled with a diet, or the idea of carrying too much weight, would probably never think about how this process works. We may eat because we're hungry, but may also have lost touch with what our food actually tastes like. We may eat because we're lonely, and have certain mental associations with food, which we unconsciously hope will take that empty feeling away. We may even eat because we're angry, and be trying to stuff that unacceptable feeling back inside us, along with our plateful of food. In any event, it is not the taste of the food luring us back, though we may believe that to be so.

Seeing the sense of taste broken down like this is helpful, I believe, because it shows that ultimately, taste is not what we believe it to be. As we will see in the next section, small changes in environment, genetics or other variables can change the way we taste forever.

Issues Affecting Taste

I have a friend I will call Herman, who was diagnosed with Cushing's Syndrome after suffering rapid weight gain for about six months, though his eating and exercise patterns hadn't changed during that time. Cushing's Syndrome is caused when the adrenal glands begin to secrete more cortisol in response to stress or other internal imbalances.

Thankfully, Herman's doctor discovered that his levels of B3 and zinc were very low, and helped them get back to normal levels with supplementation. But in the meantime, Herman had suffered nerve damage to the lingual nerve and glossopharyngeal nerve, which pass taste information to the central nervous system and the brain.

Herman had been so worried about his rapid weight gain that he had failed to notice that for months now, food hadn't tasted the same, and that he failed to derive any real enjoyment from the act of eating. After his doctor helped him label what was happening to his body, he admitted that his sense of taste had become so eroded that he had been substituting memories of what his favorite foods used to taste like. On the advice of his doctor, Herman began to supplement his diet with B3, zinc and other vitamins, and has managed to recover some of his sense of taste. With further investigation, he hopes to be back to normal soon, and to lose the weight he gained as a result of increased cortisol in his body.

Herman's story is important to a program of weight loss because it clearly illustrates how the body will carry on, by adapting to almost any situation it encounters. When his doctor first asked about his sense of taste, as a routine part of his diagnostic process, Herman couldn't remember there being a difference. But his brain had formed thoughts about food, and those thoughts were substituted during the act of eating. It starts to make sense that by becoming more aware, and more authentically "with" ourselves at every moment, we can avoid moments of unconscious substitution like this, and make healthier progress.

Herman's is not the only case in which the sense of taste can be dulled, however. Ageusia, or the complete loss of taste functions, is one very common way that taste can be affected by outside means. Hypogeusia is a partial loss of our taste function. Parageusia produces unpleasant tastes. And dysgeusia results in our inaccurately tasting something.

Additional factors influencing our ability to taste include:

• Aging
• Color and vision impairments
• Fluctuations in hormone levels
• The genetic ability to taste phenylthiocarbamide, or PTC
• Oral temperature
• Drugs and chemicals
• Lesions in the brain's temporal lobe

In short, our sense of taste is one that may be most out of our control, or so it seems. After reading these past sections, you may feel as if there's no real way to know yourself, unless you were to undergo a battery of tests. Conversely, you may only be concerned with what tastes good to you, not caring how it affects the systems of your body.

But as we will see, our sense of taste can be transformed, just as the three poisons we studied in the last chapter can be transformed into antidotes.

"Curing" with Poison

Some of you may have heard of homeopathic medicine, or seen homeopathic remedies in your local health food store. But few may understand the connections between homeopathy and trying to lose weight.

Homeopathy was developed in Germany by Christian Friedrich Samuel Hahnemann. In his own experiments, he noticed that when a poison or venom was diluted and then applied to a healthy body, it produced many of the expected symptoms. But since the body was healthy, it also developed antibodies to the poison, making it stronger in the long run. This method of treating "like with like" is similar to our current practice of vaccinations, in which we inject small amounts of a bacterium or virus capable of causing a disease, along with a measurable amount of antigen, in order to stimulate the immune system.

Our sense of taste operates in much the same way. Foods that may in fact be bad for us, by offering no real nutrition to our bodies, many times "fool" the brain into thinking it has done the right thing. Just as we adjust to small amounts of poisons injected into the bloodstream, we can also form a kind of antidote to non-nutritional foods and beverages. The message to the brain remains the same. But in the meantime, our bodies are not being adequately fed. Our energy is lowered, and our bodily systems become depressed.

Conversely, when we eat foods that serve the greater good of the body, and give it the highest levels of nutrition, we may experience surges in energy, and begin to feel the quick results many of us seek. Though many complain that broccoli doesn't taste as good as a burrito, the body experiences these foods in a completely different way. Just as the brain can be fooled into thinking that "bad" foods are good for us because of various chemical reactions, it can also help us learn to like the taste of brown rice, broccoli, or soy beans because we become addicted to the positive results we experience.

In that way, we all learn to apply the antidote, both internally, with our emotions and physical reactions, and externally, with our behaviors. This goes a long way towards transforming negative emotions, as we will see in this next section.

The Antidote to Passion

In order to bring more energy and healthier functions to our bodily systems, we need to bring the first antidote, which is awareness. Just as there is no "one size fits all" diet, perfect for anyone who wants to lose weight, there is no one way to approach the three poisons, however they manifest in our lives.

Passion, the first poison we studied in the last chapter, is also sometimes translated as *greed*. This can take the form of creating a false hunger in us, so all we want is more, more, more, without ever stopping to notice sensual things like taste, or even if our stomachs are already full. Greed may mean wanting to wear a size 2, even if it (literally) kills us, just so we can impress our friends, or just to wear expensive designer labels. It may also mean that we want to make ourselves somehow better than others, or enforce an illusionary distance between our experience and that of other people.

The natural antidote to passion and greed is generosity and, even if you're the most selfish person in the world, this can be attained with awareness. Traditional diets often use the tactic of shame to teach us when to stop eating. But that path may actually teach the opposite of what it intends, enforcing the idea that somehow, we are not worthy of being fed or nurtured. We may even come away with the idea that we must stop listening to that inner voice that tells us when it's time to push away from the table.

We may also become confused by the concept of generosity, thinking that it means we must share what we have with others. That's certainly one way to look at it. If we have more than enough food—in our homes, on our plates—we can usually afford to share. If we grow vegetables in our gardens, there are usually enough tomatoes for us and our family, as well as the elderly woman across the street. But there are other ways of looking at our passion or greed.

Greed can manifest as the desire to control one's body or environment so tightly that there's no room to be human anymore. The slightest weight gain—a pound of water retained after a workout, for instance—may send someone into a frenzy of activity and planning, trying to rid themselves of exactly what their body needs at that moment in time, which is hydration. Greed can also manifest as the desire to be perfect, despite the fact that we are all human and fallible. Only by applying the concept of generosity to ourselves, as well as the rest of the world, can we hope to break this destructive pattern.

The Antidote to Aggression

Aggression, as we have seen, can also be thought of as aversion or ill-will. Instead of examining qualities we do not want to look at in ourselves, we project them onto others, and the result is anger towards them. We want our lives to be comfortable at all times, and devoid of any suffering. When we experience difficult emotions, our first instinct is to back away from them. We try to get someone else to take them on instead, so our lives can go back to "normal." And only when the unpleasant feelings go away do we feel we've succeeded.

This often manifests in people trying to lose weight out of hatred for the body, which refuses to do our bidding. It doesn't lose weight fast enough for us. We don't look like that model in the picture. Our abs aren't sculpted enough, and no amount of crunches seem to work. We are willing to take aggressive risks, in the form of too much exercise, surgery, pills or other means, in order to achieve the prime directive of building our perfect body.

The natural antidote to aggression, therefore, is loving-kindness. This is a word that's difficult to translate from the original Sanskrit. But basically, it means to extend to oneself and others the wish that all be free of suffering. When we're applying this antidote, we wish all beings to enjoy the state of ease and wellbeing, and to be protected, safe and happy.

It does not mean that somehow, we'll be protected from ever experiencing anger, or acting aggressively in the future. These emotions are hard-wired into us for our survival, and it would be very difficult indeed to rid ourselves of them. Instead, we extend what we want for ourselves—contentment, safety and freedom from suffering—to all beings. This helps to mitigate the effects of anger, and transform it into a powerful force for change.

The Antidote to Ignorance

Ignorance, as we have seen, is a failure to understand the world as it really is. We may choose to believe what we want to happen, or just be operating in a way that's not in harmony with the other beings and circumstances around us. It is the "head in the sand" approach to anything, whether it requires expert knowledge or not. We are sure that we know more than the next person, or even the Universe itself. If only "they" would get behind our goals and plans, everything would work out fine.

Ignorance can manifest in many ways while losing weight. We see ignorance every day in the mass media, through images of ultra-thin women and men populating most of our advertisements. This tendency may be partially at fault for the rise in anorexia and other eating disorders, which people adopt in order to achieve this impossible dream.

The central question of ignorance is whether the keys to happiness, directly related to achieving our best body, can be found within us. Many of us constantly crave the attention, affection and approval of those around us. But that generally leads to frustration, when the attention or affection isn't immediately forthcoming, or even anger, if approval isn't given in the way we want. Because our bodies have been equated on some level with desirability, or the "right" to enjoy attention, affection and approval, it's not a big leap to see how the journey toward losing weight is one bound to bring this poison forward.

The natural antidote to ignorance is wisdom. If we open ourselves with awareness about the entire picture, not just the tiny part affecting us, we may see that this situation can be approached in another way, one that's healthier for all involved. It does not mean that we will suddenly be immune from frustration and anger, or that we will magically receive all the attention, affection and approval we crave. Instead, it means that we use our minds and senses to gain wisdom about a given situation.

We may be excited to start a new fad diet we've read about in a magazine. All our friends are talking about how much they've lost by following it. But if the diet includes only grapefruit and water and we're allergic to grapefruit, going on this diet is not healthy, even if it causes us to lose weight. Your mind and senses may tell you that a more balanced diet, with fruit, vegetables, grains and protein sources you're not allergic to, will yield a better result.

It does not make the diet bad, or your friends wrong for having used it. The process of transforming ignorance simply means that you find the way that works for *you*, without causing any harm to yourself or anyone else.

Meditation

Last week, our meditation sessions brought us closer to the three poisons, and began to make them a bit more personal. It's fine to read about an abstract concept like "poisons" and try to understand it. But it's another thing altogether to find a concrete way to apply this concept to your daily life. Hopefully, the relationship between the three poisons and the poisons you may inadvertently be putting into your body may have started to resonate a little.

This week, we'll take what we've learned and see how we're always capable of transforming these poisons, using certain antidotes. One antidote for losing weight may be to find a safe exercise plan. Another may be cutting back on sugary soft drinks. The important thing is not to become too rigid about what we think, but to encourage our minds to be as flexible and yet still discerning about what we experience.

It takes a good deal of practice, but this type of wisdom can be applied in many areas of your life, and can help tackle large and small problems alike.

- Begin by going into your private meditation spot and closing the door, if possible. Make sure to have your notebook and writing implement or mini-cassette recorder handy to record your experiences after the meditation. Spend a few moments just acclimating yourself to this new space you have created.

- Then bring your body into your preferred meditation posture, either seated on a mat or blanket, with your legs crossed under you, or seated in a chair, with your feet placed flat on the floor. Spend a moment or two arranging yourself into a posture that is upright and dignified, without being too tight or controlled. Try to feel your way into the pose that's right for you. Take your time. This moment is about you and your personal development.

- Next, move through the 7 Points of Posture, making sure you bring awareness to your body, and balance to your practice.

- Bring awareness to your seat and legs, making sure you have a solid foundation for your meditation.

- Next, soften your gaze, and direct your eyes about 6-8 feet in front of you, looking slightly downward.

- For the third point of posture, hold your spine upright and balanced, with the vertebra stacked one on top of the next.

- Now bring your awareness to your shoulders, making sure they're being held at the same level, with no tension.

- And then bring your awareness to your neck and throat, swallowing once and directing the neck downward to follow the gaze.

- Next, hold the tongue lightly on the roof of the mouth and leave the mouth open a little bit, which will make breathing easier.

- Lastly, hold the hands flat on the thighs or over the kneecaps, with the palms down.

- Once you have established your meditation posture, let yourself relax into it. Feel the parts of your body working together as you begin to notice your breath. Feel the breath on its complete journey as it moves in through the mouth and nose, expands through the throat, the top of the lungs, the bottom of the lungs, all the way down to the belly. Then feel the breath as it leaves the belly, the lungs, the throat and the nose and mouth again.

- Take five full breaths in and out here, just noticing your breath. When you notice a thought in your mind, say "thinking" to yourself and let the thought dissolve as you breathe out. Remember, you are not trying to chase away thoughts, or label them as "bad." Everyone has thoughts, and this exercise is simply to familiarize you with the way your mind works.

- When you feel ready, begin to connect each of your senses to your meditation. On most days, most of us walk around completely unconscious, assuming that the parts of our body will work in tandem, or that our senses will bring us the information we need in order to survive. But for the purpose of losing weight, we need to establish a new connection between our bodies and our senses, one that's a bit more intentional.

- Start with your eyes. Though your gaze will be soft and directed slightly downward to the floor, notice how your eyes are bringing you visual information. Notice the light in the room, how it may be hitting something in your field of vision, or creating shadows. Then refocus your gaze and let that go.

- Bring your attention to your ears, registering the way they feel on the side of your head, and how they filter auditory information. Notice any sounds in the room with you now, and then let them go as you breathe out.

• Do the same for your sense of smell, bringing your attention to your nose and just spending a moment there, noticing how it feels on your face. Maybe your nose is stuffed up, or perhaps you have sensitivities to certain smells. Notice how your nose works to help you register olfactory information, and then let it go, breathing out.

• Now begin to notice your mouth and tongue. Move your tongue around in your mouth a little, even it might feel weird. Notice how your tongue feels in your mouth. If you can, try to get in touch with all the tiny tastebuds there, which distinguish all the various and wonderful tastes in the world. Then let this go, breathing out.

• Keep your breath moving in and out of your body as you focus your attention on your hands, especially the sensitive skin of the palms and fingertips. This is the primary area we use to experience our sense of touch, one of our most important senses. Feel the skin register even the smallest changes in temperature in the room. Notice how the tiny hairs on the back of your hands are activated whenever a gust of air blows by, or when you move through a new environment. Then let that go and breathe out.

• Spend the next five breaths watching your breath, and labeling your thoughts as they arise in your mind. The goal is to notice your storylines, and then remind yourself to come back to the present moment before they have the chance to carry you away.

• Now bring your attention to your body. Just imagine yourself as if you're standing in front of a mirror. Notice your thoughts about your body as they move through your mind. Notice any shifts that occur as your feelings take root in your body. Does your stomach clench up at the thought of being observed? Do you start to feel light-headed or dizzy? Just notice how you look, and then how you feel about it for a few breaths.

• Notice any feelings you may have of passion, such as the desire to eat as much as you possibly can, no matter how full it makes you feel, or the desire to lose more weight, even if the person you find in the mirror is perfectly healthy.

• Notice any feelings of aggression, such as anger, that you've "let yourself go," or even anger towards your mother, who "gave you those hips in the first place."

• Notice any feelings you may have of ignorance, such as the desire to stop eating altogether, or to force yourself to go on a starvation diet as punishment for the way you look.

• Hold the image of your face and body in mind, along with any feelings it brings up in you, as you return to your Base Practice. Keep your breathing going for the next five breaths. Then let the image go as you breathe out. Come out of the meditation.

Follow Up Exercise

This can be a very powerful meditation for many people, so give yourself a little more time than usual to come out of the meditation and return to normal consciousness. If you need to, grab a glass of water and move around a bit before returning to your seat.

Then get your notebook and writing implement or cassette recorder and write or speak about your experience. Before your mind can form judgments or harden itself for or against what it has "seen," let it all come out in a rush. It doesn't even matter if you're writing or speaking in complete sentences. Just let your mind tell you what it has to say.

Often, we suffer through various states of mind caused by these three poisons because of our very well-trained defense mechanisms. We sidestep. We deny. We laugh and say it doesn't matter anyway. But your internal experiences are key to understanding your body and the way you carry yourself in the world. If that isn't crucially important to how we all live, I don't know what is.

As you write down your experiences, take a few minutes to consider these questions:

• How did you feel as you arranged yourself into your meditation posture?

- Was it easier or harder for you to run through the 7 Points of Posture?
- Could you find your way into your preferred posture without looking in a mirror?
- How did holding yourself in this way make you feel, inside and out?
- Were you able to watch your breath without too much trouble?
- When you connected each of your senses to your practice, were you able to feel reawakened and rejuvenated in each one of them?
- How does it feel to label your thoughts in meditation, and then let them go with your out breath?
- Do you find yourself labeling yourself as a bad meditator for having thoughts?
- Do some of the same thoughts come back later, and try to carry your mind away?
- When I asked you to imagine yourself in front of a mirror, just looking at your body, what was the primary feeling that came up for you?
- If there was more than one emotion, what were the others?
- How did you feel being observed like that?
- What feelings of passion were you able to identify?
- What feelings of aggression were you able to identify?
- What feelings of ignorance were you able to identify?
- Were you in a hurry to get out of this meditation?
- If so, why do you feel that might be true?
- Finally, how do you feel about yourself now (check in with your body and mind)?

Spend a few minutes answering these questions and letting your mind release all of its thoughts and feelings about this meditation. Then direct your attention inward again, just for a moment:

- How does your body feel? Are you left with any lingering sensations?
- How does your mind feel? Do you have any emotions that may be hard to let go?

Please take a moment to record your thoughts and feelings before moving on.

Off the Mat Practice

During the week (or more) you decide to practice with taste, please don't forget to do your meditation exercises every day. It may be easy to blow off meditating, saying, "Oh, I feel fine. I don't need to meditate today." But meditation isn't medicine that you take for a headache. It's an ongoing process that helps all of us learn to deal with the material in our minds, which contributes to our emotions, and subsequently, changes in our bodies. Doing it every day helps us become more familiar with ourselves. Over time, we will find ourselves on friendlier terms with our bodies.

As well, make sure to record your experiences after every session. You may find yourself excited and raring to go on some days, slow and blue on others. The one constant will always be the inner voice within you, and your ability to bring it out into the open with your actions. If you don't believe you can have any real effect on your body, this exercise will prove you wrong if you do it faithfully.

Each day during the week, make sure to bring your attention for at least sixty seconds per day to your mind and then your body. Check in to see what your real thoughts are, and how they may be coloring your reality. Check in to see what feelings you're having, and where they're lodging themselves in your body. And finally, scan through the parts of your body to make sure you're not unconsciously carrying thoughts or emotions anywhere.

Feel yourself in your body, without apologies. Know that even if you want to make some changes, you are still you, and there's no changing that. Let yourself be present in as many moments as you can during the day.

With each meal you eat, take at least one minute to fully taste the food you're eating. Take it into your mouth very slowly. Let it hit your taste buds along the tongue, and move toward the back teeth and palette. Chew each bite with your full attention, letting simple tastes, like that of a carrot, or complex tastes, like that of a French sauce, permeate this wonderful sense. Mobilize each part of your mouth in order to relish the act of eating.

When you're finished, notice how you feel, inside and out. Write or speak briefly about it, using your notebook or mini-cassette recorder.

Think about what eating means to you, in terms of taste, and how your life would be less textured if it weren't part of your experience.

Extend Your Practice with Story

Last week, you added a few paragraphs to your ongoing personal narrative. This week, we'll go a little further, looking not only at the cosmetic nature of the human body, but about how our minds can shape how we perceive and even experience our own bodies.

To begin, spend a few minutes reading over or listening to what you wrote last week. Again, re-writing is forbidden. Just look at what you wrote and know it was the truth for you at that time, even if it has changed in a week's time. If you can, see beyond the words to the feelings that person, who may not feel like you now, may have been feeling at the time.

Then think about the image you saw of yourself during your meditation session this week. If some time has passed since then, read over the notes you took immediately after the first session. Without thinking too much about it, begin to write a paragraph about the things you saw and liked about yourself. It could be the way your hair shined in the light coming through a nearby window, your beautiful smile, or even the shape of your calves. Try not to be objective, or write about how other people *might* perceive you. This exercise is about how you feel about yourself.

Many people say they can't find five things they like about the way they look. But I challenge you to find five of them. They must be external things, not personality qualities (this is another way we tend not to deal with looking at ourselves). The point is not to torture yourself but to truly look at who you are, right now, and be able to see through the things you don't like, to the positive things you may be overlooking.

After you have written a paragraph or so on the five things you like about your body, make a short list of the things you don't like. You may be tempted, as most humans are, to make the list very long, or to fill several pages with your shortcomings. But this doesn't help. Instead, limit yourself to five things you really don't like about your body. It may be your stomach, your upper arms, or even your ankles. But don't just list the body part you're not fond of; give it a reason for why it gets under your skin, so to speak. Explain why you don't like this part of your body.

Describe the way you feel because your body is like this now.

Remember, no one is listening but yourself, so resist the urge to say what you think I want to hear, or someone else in the room may want to hear. This is for you alone, so it's always best to be honest and real. When you're finished writing or speaking your words, read over what you have written, or rewind your tape to the beginning of this session and listen to what you've said, all the way through. Listen to what your inner self is saying, between the lines. Validate yourself by really paying attention to what is going on inside right now. Then put your work aside for the week.

Next week, we'll delve into the topic of satisfaction, which can sometimes resonate very strongly for people who want to achieve their best body. From the food we eat to the way we look at ourselves, we are always searching for that transcendent moment, that way to reach beyond ourselves to the divine energy we feel all around us. Satisfaction is one word we use for this very elusive quality. Until then, reward yourself for your excellent work this week. It doesn't have to be expensive, or even food-related. A bunch of hand-picked flowers, a long bath, a hike, or even a long phone call with a friend can be just the ticket to affirming our presence on the earth, and our connection to all living things.

Chapter Five

Satisfaction

Mick Jagger famously sang about not being able to get it. Countless leaders over countless centuries have fought wars trying to obtain it. And each of us gets up in the morning, renewed and rededicated to finding it for ourselves.

But satisfaction has proved to be anything but easy to obtain. Whether we're trying to lose weight, adopt a new exercise plan, or just find a meaningful job, we're trained to want the best, but settle for whatever we can get. This sends a stream of mixed messages to our minds, and can result in a severe case of confusion for most people.

The good news is that the answers lie within you.

But before we move on, let's take a moment to check in from last week:

- Did you get to do your meditation exercises every day of the week?
- If so, how did you enjoy your meditation sessions?
- If not, what stood in the way of your meditations?
- With each day, was it easier to find your way into your meditation posture?
- Were you able to use the 7 Points of Posture pretty easily?
- Do you experience any physical pain while meditating?
- If so, were you able to find an adjusted posture that worked for you?

- How did you find the process of connecting your senses to your meditation?
- Do you find your senses more activated in your daily life as a result of doing this?
- What was the first thing you noticed about yourself when you stood in front of the mirror (in the meditation)?
- What was the last thing you noticed about yourself?
- Did any strong feelings come up for you when you did this meditation?
- If so, what were they?
- Did any strong physical sensations come up for you?
- If so, what were they?
- Did you do the Follow Up Exercise and Off the Mat Practice, by recording your experiences and practicing being in your body for at least sixty seconds each day?
- If so, what was one thing you found out about yourself?
- Were you able to Extend Your Practice with Story, by adding five things you liked about what you saw when you looked in the mirror, as well as the five things you didn't like?
- Finally, did you bring your full attention to your eating, trying to taste each morsel of food you consumed during the week?

Take a few minutes while you record your answers to these questions. Feel free to write or speak about anything else that may be very strong in you now. You may still be fuming from an argument at work, or angry about an altercation with someone on the road. You may feel sad because of a recent death in the family. Just notice how you feel at this moment. Check in with your body, to see where you may be holding any feelings or tension.

If you need to, spend a few more minutes writing about whatever you've found inside. You are strengthening the connection between your mind, body and spirit as you do so.

Retaining Weight

It has long been suggested that the first person who finds a real "cure" for being overweight will become an instant millionaire. But recently, there have been several important scientific discoveries that are helping us understand the entire picture of how the body stores and retains excess weight.

The most interesting correlation involves stress, and its role in determining the shape of our bodies. Most, if not all, of us experience stress in some form. Whether we're worried about our health, our children, our spouse, mate or love life, our financial situation, or even our spiritual development, stress comes up, and begins to take a toll. It can affect our mood, making us want to lash out at those around us or curl up in a ball and cry.

But stress also affects the insides of our bodies. When we're feeling a lot of external stress, our adrenal glands are one of the first areas to be affected. Normally, they're responsible for secreting the hormone cortisol in a diurnal pattern, which helps their levels remain highest in the morning and lowest at night time. Cortisol is a very normal part of the human body, and helps to maintain blood pressure. But since it also stimulates fat and carbohydrate metabolism, and oversees the release of insulin and maintenance of blood sugar levels, keeping cortisol constant and steady becomes especially important.

Stress does anything but keep cortisol levels constant. When we feel stressed, our bodies immediately secrete excess cortisol. This interrupts the desired pattern of more cortisol in the morning and less in the evening, and seems to promote weight gain as a result of this disruption. A few studies have even found that higher cortisol levels can affect where our excess weight accumulates, usually around the belly or abdominal area. This can become problematic for some, since added belly fat has been associated with cardiovascular disease, heart attacks and strokes.

Stress is one very common way we all adjust the cortisol levels in our bodies. But Cushing's Syndrome, in which the body produces very high levels of cortisol because of a shift in brain chemistry, is another way our bodies can be affected. Along with weight gain, other symptoms of Cushing's Syndrome include upper body obesity, rounded face, increased fat around the neck, and fragile, thin skin that bruises easily, among others. Doctors have several tests they can perform which indicate the presence of Cushing's Syndrome.

Stress remains one of the most common ways of experiencing a "spike" in cortisol. However, the results are not constant among humans. Some of us are more reactive to stress, and correspondingly, our cortisol levels are likely to be higher. At the same time, stress puts all of us at a disadvantage, because we don't believe we can stick to healthy eating habits. Stress makes us crave sugar and fat, to dull the nerve endings causing us pain, and to give us the quick jolt of energy and pleasurable feelings we have when the brain releases its chemicals.

Suffering & Its Escalation

Meditation is one important way to deal with relieving stress. Among its many health benefits are:

- Breathing slows.
- Blood flow is increased, increasing exercise tolerance.
- The heart rate is lowered, promoting deeper relaxation.
- Blood pressure is lowered.
- Blood lactate is lowered, lowering anxiety levels.
- Muscle tension and headaches decrease.
- Serotonin production is increased, leading to feelings of wellbeing.
- The immune system is enhanced, assisting in post-operative healing.

All of these are wonderful health benefits. But meditation is only part of the journey.

Any study of Buddhism usually starts with the Four Noble Truths. While the Buddha sat under the bodhi tree achieving enlightenment, he was said to have made four important realizations that colored his subsequent teachings. The Four Noble Truths are:

- Life is characterized by suffering.
- Suffering derives from various origins.
- It is possible to stop suffering.
- There is a path to help stop suffering.

Usually, it's hard for Westerners to understand this concept of "suffering." The original Pali word for suffering is *dukkha*, which suggests a bit more. *Dukkha* can mean birth, aging, sickness, death, attraction and aversion, or any other way we cling to what we want, and push away what we don't want.

According to the Buddha, our lives are characterized by suffering. It is simply there, to be experienced by all at some point. Our cravings often deepen the suffering by escalating it, or keeping it going in some other way. He suggested that there is the possibility of alleviating suffering, by working with our own cravings. Usually, this is done by following the dharma (the Buddha's teachings), and his Noble Eightfold Path.

This may mean little to people who don't have a Buddhist practice. Many believe that Buddhists are serene and slightly depressed people, talking about suffering all the time and wearing strange robes. They may believe that since Buddhism is largely an Asian belief system, which has little relevance to their inescapably Western daily lives. But "suffering" is really another word to describe the state we find ourselves in when we experience stress.

When we're stressed, we want desperately to move away from whatever is hurting or irritating us, and move toward what we want to achieve, the sooner the better. We don't stop to think about what this moment may mean in the larger scope of our lives. It's annoying, and we want it to stop. Similarly, we don't want to think about aging, or death, or craving, or much of anything at all. We simply want more control over our lives than is really possible.

So the more we crave, and the more we reach for certain outcomes and push away others, the more we will suffer. Our stress levels will be higher. In fact, the more we crave, and experience attraction and aversion, the more we're really escalating our suffering. The trick to working with this very human quality is in finding how we get hooked into these reactive states, because when we give ourselves over to stress, we're making an already bad situation worse.

Shenpa

Shenpa is a Tibetan word which loosely translates as "attachment." People who have studied Buddhism for any length of time have probably heard people talking about the quality of attachment, and how it contributes to the escalation of suffering. But to leave it at that is to open the door to misunderstanding.

Buddhist teacher Pema Chodron gives a series of excellent teachings on *shenpa*, deepening the term's meaning by calling it "that sticky feeling." She draws parallels to scratching an itch, or having an uncontrollable urge to do something, even if we know it may not be the best idea for our lives in the long run. We may feel our bodies tightening when we experience it, or hear the sound of our minds snapping shut to any other alternatives. Once our minds get involved, what may have begun as an innocent slip, or even a mistake, has now taken on larger implications for us. If someone's overlooked our feelings, for example, it may not be personal. But that's how it feels—like a burning inside, desperate to turn into something tangible, like anger, hatred, frustration, greed, or some other emotion. *Shenpa*, then, can become the catalyst for a kind of mental chain reaction, which then permeates all of our interactions with others, as well as ourselves.

We have a chance, when trying to look deeper into the issues surrounding added weight, to try to work with these moments of *shenpa*. Meditation is one important tool, since it teaches us, over time, how to work with the material arising naturally from our minds. Anytime we can uproot a negative habit, like unconscious eating, "trigger" eating, or just the tendency to be overly hard on ourselves for not achieving the goals we've set, we're moving closer to a track that can bring long-term health.

Working with *shenpa* involves opening the mind, when our minds may want to do the exact opposite. For example, if someone has made a negative comment about the way we're dressed, or even made a comment subtle enough to be construed as negative, we're already in a reactive mode. We may feel a tightening in our stomach, or a little twitch in our jaw. We may just feel bad inside, and not know why it's happening. We just have a crappy feeling, about ourselves or someone else.

It is in these small moments, trapped in the cycle of attraction and aversion, when we're actually exacerbating our suffering, or stress. Because our feelings about being called "fat," for instance, are intolerably painful to us, we immediately seek to off-load those feelings. We may run to our friend's cubicle at work and need to gossip about the person who made the comment. We may call our friend or mate and go on a verbal tear. Or we may reach for the first bag of potato chips that has our name on it.

The first step in working with *shenpa* is just to notice it. All of us experience it at some point. We all have triggers from our past, or even from our present, which just bug us. When we're triggered, we can't be the "bigger" person. We become small, and sometimes, even this feeling itself becomes addictive for us. We begin to crave the drama so we can have the contented feeling of solving it. But when we notice—ah, that's *shenpa* at work—it begins to lose some of its steam, and the ability to rope us into unhealthy behaviors.

The second step in working with *shenpa* is to acknowledge it. If we can get to the point where, in the very same moment we're experiencing *shenpa*, we can see and then acknowledge it, we are capable of choosing how we react to it, rather than automatically and unconsciously reacting. This is the key difference between eating an entire box of cookies when we're not even that hungry, and choosing to have two cookies, because that will satisfy our desire for sweets.

The third step in working with *shenpa* is to find moderation, or the middle way. In the example above, receiving a negative comment may cause us to want to off-load the feeling, or even to internalize it and hurt ourselves further. But that seldom does the trick. The bad feelings still hang around, and usually we aren't happy about it. So we do something, anything, to make the painful feeling go away. We may decide to eat a box of cookies, because we associate cookies with love, with acceptance, or even just the "high" we get from our blood sugar spiking. But if we can spot *shenpa*, and acknowledge it in the moment, we also give ourselves an important choice. Sometimes, it's not about whether a food is "good" or "bad" for you. It's not carrots versus potato chips. It's giving yourself the power to make your own decisions about what's best for your body, given the goals you've set for yourself.

After all, we're not all going to be a size 4, nor should we want to be. Each of us comes into the world with a complex series of genes that make us who we are. These genetics may make it impossible, short of starving yourself, to be a size 4. So it's important to set realistic goals for *your* best body, not a super model's. Being aggressive towards yourself, by imposing starvation rations or exercising yourself to death, is just another way of increasing your suffering.

So the middle way may mean taking two cookies, or a handful of chips, or a piece of fruit, which may provide more energy in the long run. Moderation means being powerful in that moment, choosing something deliberately, and then *really* enjoying it. If you're going to have a handful of chips, chew them slowly. Revel in the crisp texture and salty flavor. Let them last as long as they possibly can.

Then notice: Did this act, of eating these chips, take away the bad feelings inside? Maybe, for a fleeting moment, when they were in your mouth and you felt like you were really doing something to take away your pain. But long-term? Probably not. Food, or exercise, or any other stimulus, doesn't have the power to take away your feelings, or really change them in any way. If you were able to seize control back, at that very moment, you succeeded in refraining from negative behavior. You robbed *shenpa*, as well as the external stimulus it drove you to, of their power over you. You reclaimed your intrinsic wisdom. You showed your strength. You proved that food, exercise and other people aren't larger than you, or stronger than you, or in control of you. In being turned upside-down, they have been revealed to be what they were all along: neutral participants in your life.

The Role of Our Senses

We all want to be satisfied. We want it in our jobs, our love lives and our relationships with our family members. We want to feel satisfied about the amount of money we make, and how we spend or save it. But when we hear or read the word *satisfaction*, the first thing that may come to mind is the act of eating.

We have seen that increased stress raises our cortisol levels, which may play havoc with our weight, no matter what shape we're in. We've seen that the Buddhist concept of suffering is analogous to our modern concept of stress. And we've seen that stress and suffering are sometimes exacerbated by *shenpa*, and the unhealthy actions we take when we become hooked by it. Awareness and acknowledgement can help us in dealing with *shenpa*, but how can we develop those qualities?

The senses play a very important role, which is why we have been connecting them to our meditation during each session. In coming back to our senses, we begin to do two crucial things. The first is that we validate ourselves in a way that's usually not done in our daily lives. And the second is that we begin to realize, perhaps for the first time, what we're *really* feeling. That may be an emotional feeling, a sensation in the body, or both.

Many of us are trained, sometimes from a young age, to lie about the way we're feeling. We learn to say that we're fine, or we're great, or we're awesome so we don't burden anyone. But sometimes, it's just not true. We all have moments of being angry, or frustrated, or scared, or disappointed. It takes a certain amount of courage to even admit this. But some of our emotions are viewed as "negative," and some are viewed as "positive." You may even know someone who says, whenever you're feeling angry, "Why are you being so negative?" So the question becomes: How are we supposed to be real about our emotions, yet deal with a society that may not be ready for them?

One important way is to factor your senses into all your activities and decisions. Rather than listening to other people's opinions all the time, what information have you been able to gather, using your sight, hearing, and senses of smell, touch and taste? For instance, if you're trying to decide whether or not to go on the grapefruit diet, which has worked so well for your best friend, think about it for a minute. *Do you even like the taste of grapefruit?*

This is a simplified example to show how we do this all the time. Rather than using the information our senses bring, in order to help us make decisions that are right for us, we allow others to make these decisions for us. That's what we're doing when we move from one fad diet to the next, looking for the magic solution that will help us stop eating, or lose weight, or want to exercise.

Meditation is one path we can use to return to the senses. Spending some time each day really feeling yourself in your body, and noticing your environment in a new way, is another. But bringing your senses directly to the source is one of the most powerful weapons you can use on the journey to achieving your best body.

Mindful Eating

Mindful eating has become a popular buzzword in recent years. But what does it really mean, especially as it applies to our daily lives?

We all eat, maybe three or four times a day, or perhaps more. Maybe we feel that we're enjoying our food just fine, thank you very much, and don't need any help from anyone else. But the act of eating has become disconnected from its original purpose, to nurture our bodies, and because of that, it deserves more of our attention here.

Eating is a completely tactile experience that utilizes all of our senses. As we're preparing the food, or even getting ready to eat it, we smell it first. The pungent aroma of spaghetti sauce filters into the room, and we're immediately looking forward to what's coming. We hear the spoon hitting the side of the pot as we stir its contents, and this sense helps us to determine how thick the sauce is. We see the beautiful red tomatoes, the whitish-yellow garlic buds, and the green basil. We feel all the textures of the ingredients as we chop them and add them to the sauce. And finally, we put the food into our mouths, savoring it, chewing it, and then swallowing.

Mindful eating begins with the notion that each of our senses is inextricably entwined as we take food into our mouths. We are eating because the experience is pleasurable. We are eating because it tastes good. We are eating because the act itself is life-affirming. Those are the sensual rewards of putting food into our mouths.

But really, we are eating because our bodies need nutrients to perform at their peak efficiency. It's easy to lose sight of this crucial fact when we're running around, trying to do our jobs, deal with stress, take care of ourselves and our families, and even make time for a few personal goals. But if we eat mindfully, choosing our food carefully from the many choices we have, preparing it with intention, and then savoring each bite as a gesture of love towards ourselves, we are not only evading the grasp of *shenpa*, we're defeating it completely.

To do this, we feel the food in our mouths, and notice the flavors as they co-mingle. We think about the things that have come together at the exact right moment so that our bodies may be nurtured by this food: the plants that gave us seeds to perpetuate their life-cycle, the people who invested their care to plant and nurture the seeds, the rain that watered them, and the people, again, who took the time to pick the fruits or vegetables from trees or plants. This is also true of animals, who also give themselves to be our food.

There are also the people who sell our food, who truck it or fly it across large distances so we may enjoy fresh fruit in winter, and even the people who work in grocery stores. They stock the shelves, they make sure outdated food is rotated out of circulation, bag the food we take home, and offer to help us out to our car if our load is too heavy.

To be truly mindful, we also need to be aware of the people who make our dishes, pots and pans, the people who transport and sell them to us. We need to thank the power company, which brings us energy so that we may cook our food. We even need to understand that we wouldn't be able to enjoy our food at all if it weren't for the natural resources of the world, which bring us this energy. If we need further evidence that we are all inextricably connected, we need look no further than the act of eating.

Lastly, mindful eating involves the concept of satisfaction. When we strive for satisfaction, we are really trying to fulfill or gratify a desire. We want to create that warm, contented feeling for ourselves, so we can feel a little more in control of our lives. We talk about satisfying our appetite, or gratifying a need. But beyond our need to eat in order to survive, we also need to create a feeling of safety. We need to feel at home in our bodies and in the world. Food and the act of eating provide the means for achieving this kind of satisfaction.

What Hooks You?

The problem, for most of us, arises when that feeling of safety and contentment does not arise as a result of our eating. *What*, we think, *this isn't supposed to happen. I govern my own life, and I say that when I eat, I get to feel good about myself.*

Sometimes it happens. You spend your time lovingly preparing a meal, then sit down to enjoy it. Perhaps that will give you a temporary feeling of wellbeing, knowing that you have taken care of your own needs. Even if you experience it, though, that feeling is bound to be short-lived, not because life is cruel but because that's the nature of our lives. We will experience a wonderful upsurge in our mood because of food (or the chemicals in food), but then we have a sugar crash. We're in a wonderful mood and decide to eat a huge hot fudge sundae, only to be miserable a few hours later, when our stomach aches.

The point is not to be bitter about the fact that life includes a wide array of emotions, but to learn to see what hooks you. Learning where you tend to experience *shenpa* can allow you to create space around it.

Instead of reacting in a knee-jerk manner the next time you have an emotional high or low, you may be able to use that extra inch or two of space to make the decision not to eat the entire sundae, or indulge in chemical-laden food that serves no nutritive purpose anyway.

But finding that spot in ourselves may be difficult, especially if you're new to meditation. If that's the case, it's usually preferable to practice with other people at first. Since we're generally looking others in the face when we speak with them, and the human face is a very expressive instrument, it's usually pretty easy for us to see *shenpa* in action. Practicing with seeing *shenpa* at work helps us to understand how we can also get hoodwinked into *shenpa*-driven behaviors.

Next time you ask a friend to borrow money, notice the way her eyes freeze up, just a little bit, like a deer in the headlights. Next time you ask your boss for a raise, notice the way his mouth purses, the teeniest amount. Or next time you ask your kids to please put their toys away, notice how their eyes glaze over.

It's not that you're invisible, or that your wishes don't matter. What you're seeing is how all of us teeter on the edge of reactivity at one time or another. We want to do the right thing, but while our brains are moving through all our options, we close down. We want to shut out whatever's causing us to experience groundlessness so that, just for a moment, we really don't know what's going to happen next. No one likes that feeling, but it's everywhere.

One last note on *shenpa*: If you're a fan of *The Three Stooges*, you'll remember a character named Shemp, who was famously afraid of everything. So if it helps you to understand this very Tibetan concept, try calling it *Shemp-a* in your mind. Shemp experienced groundlessness whenever he encountered dogs, airplanes, cars and water.

What hooks you?

Meditation

This week, our meditation will focus on understanding the link between feeling satisfied and the impermanent nature of satisfaction. After all, just as a terrible day can't last forever, a wonderful meal will not make us happy for the rest of our lives. The trick is in learning about how this happens, so that the next time it happens to you, you might enjoy an inch or two of space that helps you to make the best choices.

People who have experienced a recent loss, such as a death, layoff or romantic partner, or even a pet, may need to be extra vigilant about their emotions during this meditation. If you feel too sensitive now, too raw, come back to this exercise when you're feeling stronger, and please don't hesitate to ask for outside help from a therapist or other mental health professional if that seems necessary at this time. There is no shame in asking for help. It is a courageous act, and may facilitate speedier healing.

Since we'll be focusing on impermanence, make sure to perform these meditations when you're assured of a good chunk of "you" time. More so than in other weeks, you may need more time to unwind after this meditation, and more time to record your experiences.

- Go to your private meditation space and close the door, if possible. Know that this single act of making time for yourself is already setting you on the right path towards achieving your best body. Make sure to bring your notebook and a writing implement, or your mini-cassette recorder, if you're keeping track of your experiences in this way. Double check, to make sure your batteries are still fresh, and that the tape you're using doesn't need to be changed before you start.

- Bring yourself into your preferred meditation posture, either cross-legged on the floor, with your legs under you, or seated in a chair, with your feet flat on the floor. This week, try to find your way into the best posture for your body, without looking into a mirror. Run through the 7 Points of Posture in your mind, making sure each part of your body is supporting your practice. Adjust your body as necessary.

- As a quick reminder, the 7 Points of Posture are: the seat and legs, the eyes and gaze, the spine, the shoulders, the neck and throat, the mouth and tongue, and the hands. As you hear each "point" in your mind, bring your attention to this area. Begin to notice even subtle shifts in your body as you strive to find the best posture to support yourself.

- Now take a moment to connect each of your senses to your practice. As we have seen, our senses not only make it possible for us to take in information. They also allow us to experience the world around us in a truly sensual way. Awakening our senses results in our lives having greater meaning, because we're able to experience each moment more deeply.

- Start with the hands, bringing your attention to your palms or the tips of your fingers, whichever seem more sensitive to you. Sometimes, when we bring our attention to a place on our bodies, it may seem more alive. See if that happens to you. Just rest your attention there, noticing your sense of touch as your hands rest along your legs, on your mat, or even on the armrests of a chair. Then come back to your Base Practice for one minute, just noticing your breath and labeling your thoughts as they arise.

- Now bring your attention to your ears. Again, take a moment to notice each tiny sensation as it arises in this part of your body. Can you feel a breeze as it wafts by? Notice shifts in background noise, such as the burbling of traffic outside, or the hum of lights and electronic devices in your home. Breathe here for a few moments, just letting your sense of hearing blossom in your awareness. Then let it go, and return to your Base Practice for one minute.

- Next, bring your attention to your eyes. If you have been keeping them closed for the beginning of the meditation, open them slightly, keeping your gaze cast slightly downward, towards the floor. Notice how your eyes feel differently as you open and close them, depending on how much light is allowed in. Notice how the colors of objects are affected as your gaze changes. Stay with your sense of sight for a few more breaths, just taking it in. Then let it go, and return to your Base Practice for one minute.

- Next, bring your attention to your nose. Wrinkle it, widen and narrow the nasal passages, and feel how the tip of the nose is sensitive to the slightest changes in the atmosphere. As you connect your sense of smell to your meditation practice, become aware of how your nose is constantly serving the greater good of your body. It helps you avoid anything potentially harmful, and keeps you safe from any unwelcome intrusions. Stay with your sense of smell for a few moments, and then return to your Base Practice, watching your breath and labeling your thoughts as they arise.

• Finally, bring your attention to your mouth. Notice how the air feels against your lips, as well as your front teeth, if you have your mouth open slightly. Because this area of the body is so sensitive, you may feel tingling on your tongue, or even your lips as you bring your attention here. Move your tongue around inside your mouth, contacting the backs of your teeth, and the roof of your mouth. Stay with your sense of taste for a few breaths, and then return to your Base Practice for one minute.

• If you've had your eyes open for this part of the meditation, close them now. This usually makes it easier to visualize the guided part of the meditation. If you need to, take a moment to re-establish yourself in your meditation posture. Sometimes, opening the eyes changes the balance completely.

• When you're ready, visualize a person you like in front of you. This may be a friend, a co-worker, a mate or just someone you feel an affinity for—it doesn't matter what the relationship is. Just spend a few moments picturing this person as if he or she is standing opposite you, or is seated in a chair nearby.

• Now picture yourself asking that person for something very large—a raise, if it's your boss, a loan, if it's your friend or parent, or even an extravagant vacation, if it's a mate. Notice the look on that person's face as you make your request. Do you see any tightening in this person's jaw? Any hesitation before he or she begins to speak? Or another change? Is he or she freely giving what you're asking for?

• Now picture someone you don't care for all that much. It doesn't have to be someone you can't stand (we're not all that strong). Just choose someone who challenges you a little, or who tends to get under your skin. Now picture that person asking you for a big favor—to accompany them to a funeral, perhaps, or to take care of their child for the weekend.

• Notice, right now, any changes already happening in your body. Before you have a chance to bury them under the emotional rug, or re-name them as something else in order to keep the peace, just see what this person's request has done to your equilibrium. Does your stomach feel tighter? Is there an aching behind your eyes?

• Also notice how your emotions are affected by imaging this request from your challenging person. If you started out feeling pretty buoyant, have you become angry? Frustrated? Bitter? Tired? Or something else?

• Sit with whatever you find inside yourself for a few breaths, just validating whatever you find. Notice where you are holding any emotional information in your body. Chart any emotional shifts, so you will be able to recognize and better understand them. Let that be okay for right now.

• Then release the image of yourself and the challenging person, coming back to your breath. Watch your breath moving in and out of your body five times, labeling your thoughts and storylines as they come up, but never chasing them out in a hostile way. Allow your body to relax back into its preferred meditation posture as your breath brings all you need back into your body.

• Come out of the meditation, allowing yourself a few extra moments to adjust to waking consciousness. Move slowly as you acclimate to the pace of your regular life.

Follow Up Exercise

When you feel ready, take out your notebook and writing implement, or your mini-cassette recorder, and record your experiences from the meditation. It is very important to do this as soon as you come out of the meditation, because this is when emotions are freshest, and when physical sensations may still be producing changes in your body.

In the past, some of my students have said they don't know what to write about when they come out of their meditations. My answer is always: anything goes. If this meditation has made you mad, write about that. If you have found yourself remembering something from your past, even if it seems irrelevant to what we're talking about, or even your goal to achieve your best body, write about it. If you have a stomachache, write about that. If you're hungry, definitely write about that.

There is really no right or wrong answer, so please feel free to let it rip. Whatever wants to pour out of you, let it come. To assist you with getting started, here are a few questions you may want to consider:

- How did it feel when you settled yourself into your meditation posture?
- Does this feel natural to you, or do you struggle with trying to find it?
- If you struggle, how does that make you feel?
- Are you able to run through the 7 Points of Posture in your mind pretty easily, so you can make sure you're creating a supportive posture?
- How did it feel to connect each of your senses to your meditation?
- When you brought your attention to each of your senses, did they seem to become a little more alive?
- Have you had any potent memories surrounding any of your senses this week?
- Have you noticed any significant emotional shifts when doing your meditation exercises?
- Have you noticed any physical changes, either internally or externally?
- When you visualized yourself talking with a friendly person, how did you feel?
- Did you notice any shifts in your emotions or body?
- What changes did you see in this person when you asked for a favor?
- How did seeing that change make you feel?
- Did you notice any physical changes as a result of this?

- Was it easy to visualize a challenging person?
- When you did, how did you feel?
- When this person asked you for a favor, what changes did you notice in yourself?
- Was there an emotional shift inside you?
- Was there a physical shift?
- If so, where was it centered in your body?
- Finally, how are you feeling now, both emotionally and physically?

For each day of the week (or more) you decide to work with satisfaction and *shenpa*, please do this meditation exercise every day. It may seem hard to carve time out for yourself, or even selfish, when in fact it's really anything but. If you are a conscious person, who wants to do the maximum amount of good in the world during his or her lifetime, you need to keep your body, mind and soul healthy and functioning. Meditation and self-knowledge helps you to do that, perhaps better than any other way we currently have. This practice, along with the act of writing down your thoughts, emotions and experiences, has been successful for most of my previous students, and I believe it will be helpful for you as well.

Off the Mat Practice

This week, when you're busy with your work and your relationships, your responsibilities and dreams, make sure to take a little part of each day to notice yourself in your body. Really getting comfortable with feeling how it is to be inside yourself may make some of us want to run for the nearest candy bar, but try to stay with it. Staying with difficult emotions, such as shame, can be a very courageous way to face the fear of failing. This process is also instrumental in transforming negative emotions into positive results.

As well, take the time to experiment with *shenpa*, a little bit each day. You don't necessarily have to go out of your way to provoke a reaction from someone. Just noticing the tiny hesitation as someone struggles with his or her emotions, or the ever-so-slight way someone's eyes glaze over when they don't want to do something, is wonderful. If you want to take it an extra step, try noticing it in yourself at least once each day, even if it's as tiny as not wanting to take out the garbage because it's cold outside.

Also try noticing how you open up or close down around food, or the concept of eating. Begin to notice your thought patterns around food. Do you finish breakfast only to begin thinking about lunch, still hours away? Do you fantasize about what you will order off the menu, not even allowing yourself the pleasure of considering other options once you get to the restaurant? When you begin eating, does your mind stay engaged on the food in front of you, or does it go someplace else, spinning a story or recalling a memory?

Spend about 5-10 minutes each day noticing your thoughts, feelings and behaviors around food. Then write about what you've discovered, making sure to include any feelings that came up strongly, as well as where they might have been located in your body.

Extend Your Practice with Story

Last week, you added a few paragraphs to your personal narrative, providing five things you liked about yourself when you looked in the mirror, and five things you didn't like as much. When you're ready to get started, read over what you wrote last week. Does it still seem like the way you feel now? If not, why do you think your opinion has changed?

Without changing anything you wrote, just read it over one more time, bearing witness to the person you were last week, and the person you are today. Then think about your interactions with other people recently. Maybe you work in an office, and see people all the time. Or maybe you are a stay-at-home mom, without much contact outside of your children. But think about the last time you interacted with an adult.

Were you aware of how that person may have perceived you physically? Did you invent a storyline about it in your mind, or even say or do something funny, to deflect from the shame you may have been feeling at the time?

Once you've gotten in touch with that moment in your life, spend a few minutes writing about it. Make sure to include as many details as you can: what you were wearing, what the other person was wearing, where the conversation or interaction took place. Include interior moments, telling about how you felt when you saw this person, and even how you wanted this person to perceive you. Put in how you felt you looked at that time, whether you had an authentic awareness of your body, or whether your mind filled in what it had invented about your physical stature.

When you've finished about a paragraph or two, write a little more about how the person you were talking with seemed to accept or not accept you, based upon your size or weight. Did he or she say anything, or do anything to make you feel welcome? Unwelcome? Approved of? Disapproved of? Were any harsh words exchanged, or did your interaction with this person seem calm and above-board?

Lastly, take a moment to write one last paragraph about how you wanted that person to react to you. Put some serious thought into it, and don't be afraid if your mind comes up with something embarrassing. Maybe at that moment you really did want your boss to hug you and give you some encouragement, because you'd had a hard day. Maybe you hoped that your landlord would notice how hard you've been working and give you a little leniency with the rent. Whatever you find, go with it. This is very fertile territory for people wanting to reshape their bodies, because reshaping the body often means that first we must reshape our minds, along with our attitudes toward ourselves, which we may be projecting into the world.

When you're finished, take a moment to re-read what you have written, or rewind the tape and listen to what you have said. Again, resist the urge to edit your feelings. We all do it, so they might sound better to some Internal Editor, but this is counter-productive. The first thing that comes out of your mind or mouth will probably be what you mean anyway, so there's no use in changing it now. You were that person five or ten minutes ago, and that's completely valid.

Put your work aside for the week. If you want to, please feel free to return to this exercise more than once per week. It's not necessary, but if you feel the itch, by all means come back and write a bit more about this particular interaction, or another one that may have come up in the meantime. Your storytelling practice is one very important way of seeing your own thoughts and feelings about the body you have now. In time, we'll use it to help reshape those thoughts and feelings, and to help you take actions to mirror that on an external level.

Next week, we'll focus on size and the search for self. We all derive some of our self-esteem from our size, and how acceptable or unacceptable that may be in our society. From large to small, we'll see how being a different size may effect your emotional life in ways you may not expect, and explore ways to deal with any sudden shifts in emotions as you move through the events of your weight loss journey.

Chapter Six

> "When we are young we generally estimate an opinion by the size of the person that holds it, but later we find that is an uncertain rule, for we realize that there are times when a hornet's opinion disturbs us more than an emperor's."
>
> - Mark Twain, "An Undelivered Speech," 3/25/1895

Size & the Search for Self

Whether we realize it or not, we all walk around with a very solid view of ourselves. We may believe that we're fairly mellow and agreeable, but in order to function, we're constantly classifying all the information coming at us. In order to do that, we need a very rigid hierarchical system, which our brains use to help us deal with the stimuli in our lives.

This week, we'll begin to look at the ways we are all affected whenever our size changes. It may be different for everyone, but by delving into the meditations and exercises here, you'll be well on your way toward learning what triggers your emotions.

But first, let's take a moment to check in from last week:

- Did you get to do your meditation exercises every day of the week?
- If so, what did you notice most about your meditation sessions?
- If not, what stood in the way of making time for yourself in this way?
- Each time you meditated, was it easier to find your way into your meditation posture?
- Were you able to remember the 7 Points of Posture without too much trouble?
- Do you experience any stiffness or discomfort while you were meditating?
- If so, were you able to adjust yourself without losing your concentration?

- As you connected your senses to your meditation, were you able to feel more awakened?
- Are your senses more active in your daily life?
- If so, what experiences have helped you notice this?
- When I asked you to picture a challenging person asking for a favor in your meditation, how did that make you feel?
- Were you able to notice instances of *shenpa* in yourself, as a result of this meditation?
- Did you notice any strong feelings, like anger or fear, come up for you during your meditation sessions?
- If so, what were they?
- Did you notice any strong physical sensations during this part of the meditation?
- If so, what were they?
- Were you able to bring your storytelling practice Off the Mat, by becoming more aware of yourself in your body each day?
- If so, how did it feel to notice the size, shape and weight of your body?
- Were you able to practice with mindful eating, noticing each bite, and savoring each mouthful before you swallowed?
- Did you notice any moments of *shenpa* in others this week?
- Did you notice any moments of *shenpa* in yourself, especially around food and the act of eating?
- Did you make sure to write down your feelings and reactions as a result of this practice?
- Were you able to Extend Your Practice with Story, by thinking about the last interaction you had with an adult, and then writing about expectations, worries and perceptions you may have carried into the situation?
- Did you extend your writing a bit further, to include how you wanted to be perceived?
- Finally, were you able to bring a little more overall awareness to your life this week?

Take a few moments with your notebook or mini-cassette recorder and just think about these questions. You can choose to answer them in order, or just use them as a jumping-off point for something else that may be on your mind from last week. Please don't feel constrained. If something else is burning to get out of you, by all means, write it down. But do make sure to go through all the things you did for yourself last week, and note them in this record you're keeping.

Then take a minute to check in with your mind and body. Are you having any strong feelings as a result of something in your daily life? Are you having any strong physical sensations? If so, spend a little time writing about how you find yourself today. You are learning to delve deeper and deeper into yourself from week to week, and measuring your progress with your meditations, your growing awareness, and your storytelling practice.

Building a Sense of Self

All of us need to know who we are, in order to survive. As we form our first relationships, usually with our parents, we use our senses to determine which words and behaviors are acceptable, and which are not. Infants and children develop millions of ways of telling whether or not they have gained approval. A raised eyebrow from your mother may tell you "no," in a way that never requires clarification. A warm smile from your father is immediately translated into a flood of relief inside. We know we have gained approval, and that we're safe.

The same is true when it comes to weight and size. For instance, in many cultures, it is acceptable for men to be larger than women. As providers, men are supposed to be stronger, in order to wield more physical power. As a result, male children who are slight of build may receive negative messages about their prowess in traditionally masculine arenas such as sports, hunting and warring/defending. Female children who are born larger than the societal norm may also receive negative messages. It may be assumed that they will consume more than their fair share, be lazy, or have no chance of attracting a mate unless they watch their weight.

All of these messages are accumulated inside us, from our earliest sensory memories. Sometimes, the brain absorbs these tiny messages so quickly, we aren't even conscious that it's happening. Instead, we may find ourselves behaving in a certain way because we hold an inner belief about ourselves. We may even be surprised we feel that way. And until we see the feeling in action, we may not understand how or why we allowed ourselves to believe any of it.

These messages, along with the lessons we're taught in school, the ones we learn from our parents, and the ones that come about through our own life experiences, form our sense of self. We may not walk around every day aware of this dynamic. Instead, we may rely on it to help us make important life decisions or moral choices, which inevitably make up the better part of our experience. For someone who has a tendency to carry weight, though, this may be a very different process.

One of my favorite students is a woman I will call Penelope. She is a large woman, very warm, and fascinated by everything about life. Penelope has about twenty hobbies, and displays an innate curiosity about several more. As far as she is concerned, she would need three or four parallel lives in order to experience all she wants to experience. She is always asking questions, which she says has irritated members of her family in the past, as well as some of the men in her life. Originally, she came to me to get help with a memoir she wanted to write about a summer she spent working in a home for autistic children, just after college.

The main problem was that Penelope couldn't get a grasp on the central character of the narrative—herself. When I asked her what kind of person this was, what this person liked to do, what sorts of moral decisions she might make, how she voted, etc., Penelope looked at me blankly. She could answer the questions as herself, of course, but couldn't make the leap to seeing herself as a character in a narrative.

I tried to help her make the connection that all of our lives are analogous to narratives, with main characters, supporting characters, and plots that may be anything but linear. But still, she remained frustrated. I tried again, suggesting that perhaps her life was like a movie that unfolded in a certain way that summer. Again, no go. Penelope's sense of self was being tested, and she had never been equipped with the tools she might need to measure it.

In truth, very few of us are.

The Erosion of Self

I talked to Penelope over the course of several weeks, on the phone and in person. Generally, her mood remained cheerful, but there were times that she began to doubt herself and the world around her. It was as if someone had pulled the rug out from under her. She described feeling as if nothing were the same anymore, and that aspects of her life she thought she could count on seemed thin and insubstantial.

We all go through times like this occasionally. What we thought we could count on, especially about ourselves, turn out to be untrue when they're tested by a real-world situation. The Democrat we thought we'd vote for (because we always vote that way) has had a history of ethics violations. Can we still be called a Democrat? The color red, which has always been our favorite, begins to look horrible on us when we change our hair color. Do we still like red? The job that seemed perfect after college has now become stale and boring. Were we not cut out to be an air traffic controller after all?

Part of this is due to the natural rhythms of our lives. As we age, we grow, both emotionally and spiritually. We incorporate our experiences into the fabric of our lives, and develop a greater understanding of our abilities. Our sense of self has been developed and strengthened because it has been tested again and again, as we've had to respond to life's challenges.

But sometimes, our sense of self may be built with insufficient materials, which don't hold up under pressure. For example, we may believe ourselves to be ardent lovers of cartoons, and that may well be true. But if that's all we're made of, we may face a great deal of difficulty when we're faced with universal problems such as death, disappointment, old age, and other forms of suffering. Cartoons seldom provide a moral compass, or way of coping with difficult emotions.

Through these difficult life situations, we decide who we really are. Will we take the easy way out and cheat a client if we're tested? Will we collapse under the strain of a recent death in the family, or find a way to carry on? And how will we carry ourselves as we age?

Of course it's our responsibility to maintain our sense of self as we're developing. But in many ways our society erodes our sense of self. In the interest of maintaining a healthy consumer culture, television ads may try to sell us one way of being (individualism, for example), by buying into something that's anything but (the same shirt everyone else is wearing). Generalized goals like the American Dream of owning a home may be compromised when a 40+-hour workweek won't get us anywhere near affording a mortgage. Even our families, and others who love us unconditionally, sometimes add to this erosion by asking us to be people we aren't, just so we can fit in and make things "easier" on ourselves.

People who carry extra weight have an additional burden in this scenario. They are workers like the rest of us, and suffer the same humiliations and compromises all of us suffer. They are lovers like the rest of us, and experience the same joy and rejection we all do. They are family members like the rest of us, and suffer family-related issues, as well as death, disappointment and old age. But heavy people are at a disadvantage because their weight gives others permission to make assumptions about them. Among the most popular are:

1. Fat people are lazy.
2. Fat people bring their problems on themselves.
3. Fat people should change their diets.
4. Fat people drive up health insurance premiums because they don't care for themselves properly.
5. Fat people are too stupid to make the "right" food choices.

Of course, some of these assumptions may be true of individual people, but not the entire group. However, cultural prejudice against the overweight continues. We single them out for ridicule. We make them the villains in movies. Conversely, we refuse to see them as human beings, often overlooking them for promotions, or keeping them in the background, for fear they will reflect negatively on us, our families, or our businesses.

This only causes further erosion of the self. Some heavy people report feeling extremely sensitive to the perceived insults of the world, and may retain the added weight as protection. Some may do it in defiance of what's expected. Some may have tried several methods to get on a healthier path, but found little success so far. But many, if not all, experience erosion of the self when they are confronted with prejudice, judgements and hostility. This may only drive some further away from informed choices that could lead to a healthier lifestyle.

Disappearing

Penelope is not the first of my clients to feel invisible. One day we were drinking tea when she told me about the time she was literally relegated to the back of a family photograph, while her brothers and sisters were arranged like furniture in front of her, to somehow disguise her bulk.

"It would be different if my father weren't overweight, too. But somehow, that never mattered. It was as if I were part of the family when he needed to change my size, and not part of the family whenever he needed to make an impression on someone else," she said.

I've had many other clients report variations on the same theme. If they carry extra weight, intentionally, unintentionally or in a neutral way, they are usually relegated to the back of the pack. This may mean that embarrassed parents feel they shouldn't (or can't) give an overweight child any love, as if providing the same caring attitude he or she provides for others means that they are "babying" the overweight child into staying heavy.

Many go through years carrying the added burden of others' shame, or even cooperating with their own disappearance, by dutifully blending into the scenery. Overweight children may learn to be as unobtrusive as possible, or to fade into the background by not voicing any personal needs. When this carries over into adult life, overweight people may inadvertently cooperate in not getting noticed, at work and in their personal lives. Over time, this may cost them promotions, raises, or just opportunities to gain the love and affection each of us needs.

Others may fight this process of disappearing, by experiencing a good deal of misplaced anger and frustration. They may not know, at least on a conscious level, what's causing dramatic shifts in their emotions, but they do understand that bearing added weight has something to do with it. Because of this, some people may carry extra weight as a way of underlining their presence in the world. The weight comes to define them, to delineate them from the people seeking to remold and reshape them. It is internalized as an aspect of the self, simply so the heavy person will not become part of the scenery.

Penelope put it this way, "For the longest time, all I wanted was for my father to notice that we were similar, that we had many of the same issues, at least with our bodies. I could have used an ally, but all he saw was a part of himself he didn't want to be reminded of. And he couldn't get rid of me."

Ultimately, the connection between weight and disappearing depends on who you are, and how you deal with challenges to your sense of self. As with other personal issues, the "secret" lies in being as aware as possible, of yourself and your reactions, as well as what others may be seeking from you during each interaction. After all, what kind of person strives to reshape another separate, sovereign person's body? Usually, it's an extremely insecure person, who needs to control everything in his or her world to build a perceived sense of security, or a person so unused to dealing with reality that they need to project their disowned feelings onto others.

Losing the Weight, Losing the Self

So what's a person to do, to stop others from eroding their sense of self? How can each of us, in an increasingly hostile and judgmental world, keep societal "norms" from appropriating little parts of us?

The short answer is that none of us is likely to ever have complete power over the rest of the world. Therefore, it's best to develop tools and strategies to use while losing weight, beginning to exercise, or undergoing another type of program. Meditation is one very important tool to facilitate this awareness. Combined with Follow Up, Off the Mat and Story Extension exercises, meditation can heighten your relationship with yourself, so you're increasingly aware of the way you operate, emotionally and physically.

During any program of losing weight, you're bound to experience moments of doubt, that you are capable of getting to where you feel is healthy, or moments of anger, because people are treating you in a completely different manner. Some people have confided that they've also experienced a good deal of fear while losing weight, especially if it's a significant amount of weight, because they feel that they're losing their sense of self, quite literally.

"Will anyone see me if I'm small?" they ask.

"Will anyone hear me?"

"Maybe I won't seem like me anymore."

"Maybe no one will recognize me."

"What happens then?"

Each of us has a very distinct and concrete vision of who we are, and this seldom changes with time. Human beings have a knack for wanting to solidify their experiences, probably to orient themselves in an ever-changing world, and to fend off the idea of death. On some level, we may believe that our bodies will last forever, even though we know on an intellectual level that we all die sometime. Seeing ourselves for who we really are, under the flesh and social accretions of personality, keeps our sense of self intact as we endeavor to achieve the physical body that makes us happiest, and facilitates our highest functioning.

Meditation

This week, our meditation will concentrate on how our innate sense of self can either help or hinder a weight loss program. You may feel you know yourself pretty well, and perhaps you do, but it's my guess that all of us, pretty much without exception, could use some help when it comes to knowing how our sense of self is affected when our physical size changes. Preparing yourself with the tools below can help you navigate the challenging times, when you may feel under attack from the outside world.

If you have recently lost a good deal of weight, these exercises can also help with the confused emotions that can arise when you find that others are treating you in an entirely new way. You may experience fear, that you will regain the weight, or even anger, that no one treated you this well before, despite the fact that you were the same person inside. Whatever the case, be vigilant and authentic with what you find.

As always, make sure to leave yourself plenty of time after the meditation to record your experiences. The further we move into this program, the more memories you're likely to uncover.

- Make your way to your preferred meditation space, making sure to close the door for privacy, if possible. Bring your notebook and writing implement, or your mini-cassette recorder, if you've chosen to record your experiences in this way. If you've chosen the latter method, make sure your tape doesn't need to be changed or flipped over before you begin.

- Arrange your body into your meditation posture. You may choose to sit cross-legged on the floor or on a mat of some kind, or seat yourself in a chair, with your feet flat on the floor. Again, try to move the parts of your body into complete balance with one another. Without using a mirror to see yourself, feel your way into the posture that's best for your body.

- Mentally, move through the 7 Points of Posture, making sure each one is supporting your meditation in the best way possible. To remind you, the 7 Points of Posture are: the seats and legs, the eyes and gaze, the spine, the shoulders, the neck and throat, the mouth and tongue, and the hands. As you bear each point of posture in mind, make subtle adjustments to your posture, until you have achieved perfect support.

- When you feel comfortably balanced and dignified in your meditation posture, take a moment to connect each of your senses. This will help you become increasingly aware of the wholly unique way you process and filter information that comes to you. Bring your attention to each of your senses in turn: the ears, the eyes, the nose, the mouth and the hands, taking a brief moment to acknowledge how each of them are currently connecting your mind and body together.

- When you've connected each of your senses to your meditation, return to your Base Practice, taking five full, even breaths in and out. If thoughts or storylines arise, do not chase them away. Simply notice them and then touch them lightly, as if with a feather and say, "thinking" to yourself. Allow the thought or storyline to dissipate as you breathe out.

- By now, you're probably feeling very relaxed. Unless you're tired, chances are your mind is very alert. Feel yourself in your body as it is now. Take a quick look through all the parts of your body, from the top to the bottom, and see if you're holding any tension anywhere. Acknowledge whatever you find.

- Now close your eyes, in order to facilitate the next portion of the meditation. Take a moment to re-establish and re-balance your meditation posture, if needed.

- When you're ready, bring to mind a mental image of yourself. It can be yourself now, yourself as a younger person, or even yourself as a child, but it should **not** be an image of yourself in the future.

- When you have the image in mind, simply hold it there as you continue breathing slowly and evenly. Notice how you look to yourself. Notice what the first thought or feeling is when you see your image. Is it positive or negative? Do you like looking at your own image, or does it make you cringe?

- Now notice any changes in your body as you hold your image in mind. Does your heart start to beat faster? Does your stomach rumble? Do you experience an aching behind your eyes? Or something else entirely? Do a complete check of your body as you continue to hold this mental image of yourself.

- Imagine someone else is seeing this image you have in front of you now. What conclusions might that person draw about the kind of person you are? For a few seconds just keep looking at your own image while trying to imagine what someone else, who doesn't already know you, might conclude about you from this image.

- Now, while continuing to hold the image of yourself in mind, begin to see yourself shrinking. Your head becomes a bit smaller, your arms and torso becomes smaller, your hips, thighs and legs become smaller. Your feet are smaller, and so are your hands. Gradually, each part of you is re-formed as it becomes smaller.

- When your image stops becoming smaller, hold this new image of yourself in mind. First begin to notice how you feel about it. Without thinking about, be honest. What is the first thought or feeling that comes up when you see this new image of yourself? What is the thought or feeling that comes right after this one?

- Now begin to notice where your feelings are clustered in your body. Does your stomach still have a rumbling sensation? Is your heart still beating faster? Is there still an aching sensation behind your eyes? Notice your body. Notice where any feelings or thoughts may be making themselves a part of your physical experience, without trying to do anything about it.

• When you have finished checking through all the parts of your body to see if anything may be sticking around or making you feel tighter, imagine someone else seeing the image you have in front of you now. Make sure this is a person who doesn't know you already. What conclusions might this person draw about the kind of person you are, based on the image he or she can see? How might this person's treatment of you change in accordance with this "new you"?

• When you're ready, release the image of the other person, and then the image of yourself. Return to your Base Practice, slowly breathing in and out. If you notice any thoughts or storylines creeping into your meditation, saying "thinking" to yourself, and let them dissipate on your out breath.

• Come out of the meditation. Let yourself have a few extra moments to return to normal consciousness. Move carefully as you return to the sights and sounds of your waking life.

Follow Up Exercise

Before you forget about the details of your meditation, get your notebook and writing implement or mini-cassette recorder, and begin to record your experience. Emotions and thoughts may still be very vivid in your consciousness, so make sure to do this right away.

If your thoughts begin to flow, by all means, follow them. Write about what is freshest in your mind right now, because usually, you need to do this. Meditation gives you the forum in which to express these dormant feelings, along with the permission to let these thoughts out. If the pace of your thoughts or the severity of your feelings frightens you, know that in this format, expressing them is very safe. If you are angry, for example, you're far less likely to hurt anyone by writing about your feelings than if you'd decided to act out of that very hurt or angry place.

As always, if you have made any important connections, linking a present emotion to a memory, for example, make sure to spend extra time on that connection. Meditation is a wonderful way to watch your mind, and watching your mind often encourages "buried" or forgotten experiences to make themselves known again.

If you need some help in getting started, here are a few prompts:

- Was it easy for you to find your way into your meditation posture?
- If so, why?
- If not, is there another way you can learn to hold yourself, so you're not in pain, or distracted in some other way?
- Were you able to settle into a "smooth" meditation session?
- If not, did you notice any feelings you had about this exercise, this chapter, or meditation in general?
- Do you find that you can remember the 7 Points of Posture?
- If not, is there another way you can remember to check through your body, to make sure each part is perfectly balanced?
- When you connect your senses to the meditation, do you notice any particular thoughts or feelings coming up again and again?
- Do you notice that by connecting your senses to your meditation, your senses are more "alive" during your waking life as well?
- If so, have you been enjoying your senses more and more?
- Have you begun to experience the world a little more vividly?
- Have any memories come up for you, either in this meditation session, or during the days you practiced this week?
- What emotions were strongest during this meditation?
- Where did your emotions seem to reside in your body?
- What were the primary physical sensations that came up for you?
- Was it easy to "see" yourself in your mind's eye, or not?
- What was the first thought or feeling that came into your mind when you saw yourself? What was the second?
- Were you able to be honest with your feelings when you saw yourself?
- As you began to shrink yourself down, how did you feel? What was the first thing that entered your mind when you saw yourself this way?
- When you began to shrink in the meditation, did you notice any shifts in your body? If so, what were they?
- When you imagined someone else seeing you for the first time, how did that feel for you?
- Where were the feelings clustered in your body? Could you bring your attention to this place?
- How did it feel to have someone who doesn't know you look at you for the first time?

- What did you imagine that person thought about you, based upon the way you looked?
- How do you feel that person would treat you if you were your regular size?
- How do you feel that person would treat you if you were your shrunken size?
- Finally, what feelings were left in you when you came out of the meditation? And how are you feeling now?

As you get deeper into this program, it's important to do your meditation exercises every day of the week, even if you only have five minutes to spare. Making this time for yourself is an act of protest, against the way things are now, and the way things may have been for a long time. Getting to know your mind is an important tool you will use not only to assist in losing weight, but at work, in your personal relationships, and even in situations you may not even be able to imagine right now.

Off the Mat Practice

Please keep up the practice of noticing yourself in your body, at least once per day that you choose to practice with Size and the Search for Self. If you can extend this a little and stay with yourself in your body for ten minutes, or twenty, or thirty, that's wonderful. The more you can learn to live inside the body you have now, the more you will be able to treat it with compassion.

Also, while noticing yourself in your body, and how that feels to you, also take a few minutes to get in touch with the ways you may be building or eroding your own sense of self. For instance, do you refer to yourself as "a Burger King girl" while talking to friends? Do you describe all the bad aspects of your recent vacation first, so as not to make anyone else jealous? Is there a split second when you doubt what you're about to say, right before you say it?

Begin to notice these little moments. Notice how you feel right after you notice them, and how that feeling may or may not make itself known in your body. If you can, watch carefully when you experience feelings of hunger, or are in the act of eating. Try noticing the thoughts or feelings you have right before, if possible, and then right after.

If you're in the act of eating, try to notice if you have any particular associations with what you're eating. Most of us are familiar with the concept of comfort food, which is usually eaten more for the associations we may have for it, rather than for its taste. Macaroni and cheese is like this for some people. It's tomato soup and grilled cheese for others.

Are you eating for the taste of your food? For the memories and associations you have with it? Or because food makes you feel safe and protected in an unsure world?

Always, always notice, as much as you can.

Extend Your Practice with Story

Last week, you continued with your story practice, by adding a few more paragraphs to the personal narrative you're creating. In it, you thought about your last adult interaction, then wrote about how you felt about yourself, as a person in your body, and how you thought you were perceived by others. You also included how you wanted to be perceived.

Before starting on this week's exercise, read over what you've written so far, from beginning to end. You'll probably have about 10-20 paragraphs, and maybe more, depending on how inspired you've been in weeks past. Take your time. Savor each moment, each image, each memory. This is your story, and it deserves special attention.

Then think about what you wrote for a few minutes. Does it still represent the way you feel? If not, what's come along to influence the way you see yourself?

Don't change anything you wrote, even if you find a spelling mistake. One more time, read over what you've written. Try to imagine yourself as the person you were six weeks ago, four weeks ago, two weeks ago, and even last week. Be compassionate towards that person, even if he or she doesn't feel like the "you" you are today. Then find a space to continue your personal narrative, right underneath your previous work, on a fresh page.

Think about yourself as a child. Try to remember the very first time you became aware of your size and shape, relative to that of other people. What kinds of feelings do you remember having about yourself? If you can, remember the clothes you wore. Remember the feeling of pulling those clothes over your body. Remember how moving around in your skin felt, as you ran, walked, jumped or hopped.

Before your Internal Editor can stop you, put your pen to paper and start writing. Choose one particular moment from your childhood, if applicable, or from your life as person younger than you are today. Take off from there.

Do you remember receiving any particular messages from other people, relative to your shape and size? Were the messages positive or negative? Did any of them revolve around food and eating? Or were they just about your size and shape in general?

Once you've written down a paragraph or two about that particular moment, branch out a bit. Think about what methods your family used to solidify itself as a unit. This may have come in an "us against them" kind of attitude, or even in your mom or dad's way of defining your family as different from, or better than, other families. More rarely, this may have come as a message about how your family was worse than others'.

Write another paragraph about your family at the time of that memory you captured. What was the dynamic among you? Did your parents fall into specific roles, or were they more free form? What about siblings, and your relationships to them? When and where did you feel most safe as a child or younger person?

Keep writing, anything you can think of. Keep your pencil moving. If you are recording your experiences or memories with a mini-cassette recorder, stop speaking if you need to, but keep pushing yourself to dig deeper into your thoughts, even if there are a lot of "ums" and "ahs" as you pause to collect them. It may feel weird to be speaking into a tape recorder as you sit in a room by yourself, but try to think of it as a good friend, to whom you're confessing all your oldest secrets.

Lastly, think about your life now. Do you think you have carried on the traditions and methods of self-identification as your family? If so, are you comfortable with them? If not, what played into your decision to break with this way of being?

When you're finished, you should have about 4-5 paragraphs, or maybe more. There may be a little more story inside you, but when you feel that you've done all you can do at this time, put down your pen or press the stop button on your mini-cassette recorder. Take a breath.

Chapter Six

Then take a moment to re-read what you've written, or rewind your tape recorder to the place where you began.

Do not edit, no matter how harshly you may see yourself, your feelings or your words. The point is to listen to who you are right now, perhaps in a way you have never enjoyed from anyone before. In order to find success in co-mingling the goals of your mind and body together, you may need to bear witness to painful memories, ugly feelings, or even hateful thoughts about your own body. This is one very potent way to stare them in the face and force them to disappear for good.

When you're finished re-reading your work or listening to your recording, put it aside. Try to take with you the knowledge that you are a storyteller now, and you have willingly (and capably) taken on the mantle entrusted to very few people in our history.

If the mood strikes you, feel free to return to your notebook or mini-cassette recorder and add to this personal narrative during the week. You may find that the more you work with story, and get over any insecurities you may have, the more you are drawn to the act of telling your own. Write it down or record it, especially if powerful memories come up.

Next week, we'll explore the concept of emptiness as it relates to losing weight and achieving the body that's best for you. Just as no one diet or exercise plan is right for everyone, no one way of looking at the mind-body connection will resonate with every person. We'll look at how fear can keep us heavy, even if that's the last thing we want, and learn techniques to keep us from subverting ourselves to the needs of others, whether perceived or spoken. Lastly, we'll refocus our intentions from the beginning of this program, and make sure you're well on your way to the kind of success you've imagined.

123

Chapter Seven

> "The greatest fear in life is to see the emptiness
> in front of you. The greatest courage is to step
> forward and fill it with the best you have to offer."
>
> - Pierre Teilhard de Chardin

Emptiness

One of the greatest fears of most people carrying extra weight, aside from ridicule about their size, may be the fear of being empty. This may be quiet literal, meaning they're afraid of not having what they need in order to sustain themselves, including food. But it can also have other implications, relative to our thoughts and emotions, which may have the inadvertent effect of keeping us heavy, despite our best efforts to lose weight.

This week, we'll work on digging underneath some of the most common fears that people losing weight tend to feel. While each person will no doubt experience all kinds of conscious and unconscious fears during this process, depending on their background and level of sensitivity, most of us are connected in the very human way we interpret messages from our families and cultures. If we start there, we are likely to find very fertile ground.

But before we start, let's take a moment to check in from last week:

- Were you able to stick to your schedule of meditating at least once each day?
- If you had to use one word to describe your meditation sessions during this week, what would it be?
- Why did that word seem like the best one to describe your meditations?

- Has it become easier to make time for yourself each week?
- If not, what obstacles still stand in your way?
- In the weeks you've been meditating, have you found that your meditation posture is more natural?
- Did you remember to run though each part of your body as you're settling into your meditation posture, to make sure it's supporting your practice with balance?
- If you feel unbalanced in your meditation posture, are you able to make some on the spot adjustments so you're more comfortable and supported?
- When you connected your senses to your meditation this week, which sense did you notice was more awake than any of the others?
- How did you notice that this one was most awakened?
- When you saw the image of yourself as you are now, how were your feelings triggered?
- Do you remember having one feeling above all others?
- Were your feelings clustered in one particular area of your body?
- When I asked you to visualize yourself shrinking in size, how were your feelings triggered? What feeling came up most strongly for you?
- Do you remember how your feelings affected the various parts of your body?
- If you were to be as honest as possible, what did you think of yourself when you saw yourself shrunken down in size?
- In your Off the Mat Practice, were you able to notice yourself in your body a little more each day?
- Were you able to identify moments when you consciously defined yourself?
- Were you able to notice how you were drawn to food and the act of eating? If so, what were the feelings you had most prevalently?
- Did you notice any emotional associations you have with certain foods?
- When you Extended Your Practice with Story last week, did you get in touch with your first memories of being "different" because of your size or shape?
- Could you identify the ways in which your family defined itself?
- And finally, have you chosen to carry on these family traditions? Or have you decided to define yourself differently?

Remember to turn off the Internal Editor as you write down the answers to these questions, along with anything else that may be on your mind right now. If you've had a bad day at work, write it down. If you feel like eating a huge meal, write that down. And if you want to cry because you don't know how you're going to change your life, write about that. Just keep writing, or speaking into your mini-cassette recorder. Don't stop speaking or writing until you get to the end of the list, or until your mind has run out of things to say. If you need to, take a break and come back to write down the rest.

When you're finished, put down your pen or recorder and sit with the feelings you have. More than likely, it has become easier for you to look inside yourself and identify what types of feelings you're having, and where they might be sticking around in your body. Whatever you find now, take the time to validate it, writing about it if necessary. Your mind is a valuable ally, and can reveal a great deal, if you learn to listen carefully.

Fear of Nothingness

All of us are afraid of starving to death. It doesn't matter if we're large or small-framed, heavy or thin. Each of us knows, on some hidden inside level, that if we don't eat, we will cease to exist, and that's why obesity, food and losing weight comprise one of our most emotionally loaded issues today.

We're all afraid of becoming smaller and less visible. As infants, we know, even before we begin to form words and sentences, that if we notice an adult's attention straying, we can always cry. We know that if all else fails, we can use this universal signal, which draws others to us. If we can make our selves larger through noise, we can ensure our survival.

As we grow, these primordial fears seldom leave us, though they may be subsumed to our practical adults needs and wishes. We're rarely very far away from these fears, however, at least on an emotional level. Each day, we walk around in abject fear, that we will not have enough money to pay our bills and buy groceries, that we will not be able to afford adequate shelter, and that when we're old, we will not be able to fend for ourselves. We may even be driven to take risks, work at substandard jobs, or accept emotional punishment from others to make sure we have enough to eat. After all, it's this fuel that provides the energy for our daily work.

Similar fears are often released when people lose weight. Since many believe weight to be a covering, like armor, over sensitive emotional places, it's not difficult to deduce that when this weight begins to come off, old issues the weight has been covering will begin to reveal themselves again. That may be why weight is often so stubborn for us to lose, or why weight seems to come back so quickly after it's been lost.

If we exist in a defensive position, and most of us do in some way, we may be afraid of the nothingness that can come when we envision ourselves as smaller beings. If we take a lot of emotional heat from an unstable boss, for instance, we may believe that we're literally being worn away when we lose weight. This may make it nearly impossible to succeed.

If we're engaged in unsupportive or even abusive relationships, we may know, just as we knew as infants, that the only way to survive is to have a bigger self. Though we may say we want to lose weight, exercise more, or just adopt healthier choices, our circumstances may work against us. This, too, is not conducive to achieving our goals.

None of us will ever be able to exert control over everything that touches our lives, directly or indirectly. So how are we supposed to achieve our best bodies when the world is sometimes unhelpful? How can we conduct ourselves with the greatest dignity and balance in a sometimes-psychotic environment?

How Our Minds Exacerbate Suffering

While it's true we can't control everything around us, we can begin to understand how we take part in forming our own reality. The process is not magic. It's not as if we have a thought and then whatever we've thought pops magically into being. If so, "reality" would be a hilarious, Terry Gilliam universe, with dream creatures flying through the air, and people running amok as the desire for pleasure overtook any need to observe the rational mind.

In order to achieve any goal, whether it's losing weight or getting a new job, we have to start with the mind. The mind is where our electrical and chemical impulses interact to become brainwaves and signals that move to our cells, limbs and organs to promote movement. This conscious part of our being provides the framework for all we want to achieve, as well as the mental planning which needs to go into making any substantial change.

Our mind is also the seat of our stories. So while we may not be able to control our external reality, we *can* learn to tame our minds, as well as channel the power of storytelling in order to effect the kinds of changes we want to see in our lives. Even learning to observe our stories, and redirect that energy outward, as you may have already seen, will result in palpable transformation.

The reason it's crucial to get a handle on the way we're using stories is because our minds have a natural inclination to exacerbate our suffering. Suffering here is not meant as excruciating agony. It's merely the very human way we all have of making things worse on ourselves when things don't go our way. Disappointment happens, for instance, when we feel that something has been taken from us. But the anger we feel is not enough. Rather, it's often turned inward, hurting us even more than the original slight. The same is true of the other human emotions we experience.

In short, observing our stories, as well as any other stuff our minds produce, puts us in a powerful position to achieve change. By carving out this inch of space for ourselves, we are a lot less likely to become reactive, and hurl ourselves off our chosen path. By not becoming reactive, we save ourselves from truly ugly emotional territory. And by recognizing the power of our stories, we take hold of the only tool we have that is uniquely ours, and can work for us in a way that will not work for others.

Giving Up the Ghost

Humans have a unique capacity for suffering. In fact, the Buddha's First Noble Truth said that suffering is our natural way of life. Birth, death, sickness and old age are just a few of the ways we all will experience suffering in our lives. But instead of giving in on an emotional level, and getting depressed about the inevitable, we can adopt tactics that help us to cope with our day-to-day reality while providing a platform from which to develop awareness.

I look at our hopes as little ghosts, ephemeral and insubstantial. When we make a plan, it's said that God laughs. Even still, our hopes circle around our aspiration of the moment, whether it's attracting a new mate, or getting a book deal, or baking a better red velvet cake than any of our other relatives. Like us, our hopes try to solidify themselves and gain ground. They don't realize they're little ghosts floating around in the air; they just want to be real.

If we achieve our aims, we assume it's because we're good people, because we deserved it, or because we did something right in a previous life. But if we don't, we agonize over the reasons why not. Are we really bad people, but just don't realize it? Do we not deserve to have the things we desire? Did we do something terrible in a past life? This is exacerbating our suffering, because our minds are not helping us heal and move on. By following this line of thinking, we make sure that we can't move forward, because we've set our feet in concrete.

When we're trying to find the body for us, we're bound to set lots of goals. We may want to eat a certain number of calories each day, or do a certain number of crunches before work, or lose a certain number of pounds before a particular date. What we're doing is setting a desired outcome to the problem as we see it.

Part of this can be helpful. We need to see a problem before we set intentions to overcome it. We need intentions before we can take well-considered action. But whenever we focus unduly on the outcome, we can get tripped up.

This is where people usually start to scratch their heads and say, "*What?* I thought losing weight was a good thing."

Of course, setting goals and taking steps to achieve them is a good thing. This is how we make life interesting, and keep our lives vibrant and growing. It's also how we end up meeting many, if not most, of our practical needs. But when we fixate on a particular outcome, not allowing for variables such as timing, willpower or the complicity of others, we begin to sow the seeds of suffering, because we can't control what will happen next.

If you're reading this book, chances are you want to lose weight, begin an exercise program, and achieve your best body. One important secret to success lies in having intentions and making plans of action, but without investing so much of ourselves that, in the event we don't achieve what we want, we don't destroy our emotional lives. Most of us will probably remember a time when we really wanted something—a bike, a good grade, a sexy look from the object of our desire—and then what it felt like not to get that very thing, at least in the time-frame we had in mind. It can be very crushing.

Losing weight is no different. In fact, it's even more treacherous territory, because issues of survival and how accepted we are by our community, which go to the deepest parts of our being, tend to come up when we take these journeys. For now, it's enough to become cognizant of the myriad ways we become involved in storytelling episodes, which can lead to or exacerbate suffering. In time, your developing awareness will be able to discern even subtler versions of these storylines, until you're capable of directing this energy at will.

If we are supposed to make intentions, take actions and achieve goals, how can we do that without exacerbating suffering? The key is in letting go of your chosen outcome, without giving up completely.

True Emptiness

When we think about losing weight and the concept of emptiness, it always relates to the stomach, or how much food is going into the body. It may also relate to how "full" we feel at different times of the day, and different stages of our lives. However, thinking about emptiness in the spiritual sense, and applying it to weight loss, can help to clarify confusion.

A common stumbling block for many is the age-old conundrum: How do I stay true to my spiritual path and still strive to obtain goals? How can I be emotionally healthy, by moving consciously towards the things I want to achieve, while not driving myself crazy?

Buddhists have a more complex definition of emptiness, which varies from school to school, and from lineage to lineage. It is often equated with the concept of non-attachment, which people often take to mean detachment. That's where confusion sets in. It's damn near impossible to get anything done if you're detached from reality. Losing weight requires an extraordinary level of dedication, not just to making changes to one's food intake, but to dealing with the mental and emotional transformation which occurs as a result. To not engage with this process is to doom it to failure before it even begins.

When thinking about how emptiness might shed a little wisdom on the process of achieving our best bodies, I like to connect it to stress. This is a concept most people can relate to, in our sleep-deprived world. As I mentioned earlier, suffering is a kind of stress in the mind, or a disturbance that can either help us accept events as they exist, or invent fictions around them. Emptiness is the tool that helps us be present with whatever is occurring, even if we can't do much about it.

Emptiness doesn't mean rising above something, or becoming too cool and detached to have to deal with it. It doesn't mean that we're so spiritually ascended that we don't have the petty emotional concerns of mortals anymore. And it doesn't mean emptying ourselves and living ascetic, monk-like lives. Emptiness, or non-attachment, is a way of curtailing our reactivity so that we can make way for success to arrive.

About a year ago, I had a student named Will, who was sick of being heavy. He didn't care how long it took and he didn't care what he had to do—he just wanted to stop feeling so slow and lethargic. At the same time, I noticed that Will's mind was very quick. He could solve the *New York Times* crossword puzzle in about an hour (it took longer on Sundays, he told me), and had a very quick wit. His body, however, didn't go with his vision of himself in his mind. He actually became frustrated with this part of himself that couldn't "keep up" with the rest.

When Will began meditating, everything he feared rose up, seemingly at one time. Maybe he wasn't as smart as he thought. Maybe his body really ruled him, and always had. Maybe he would never achieve the kind of success he wanted as a joke writer. Maybe it was true that only his family members loved him, and only because they had to.

Will came to me, shaking, and asked if there wasn't something wrong. "Isn't meditation supposed to be calming?" He asked. "I dread every minute I sit on the cushion."

I told him that meditation could have calming and restorative properties, which were mostly felt in the organs and tissues of the body. However, because the mind is a separate entity altogether, it has its own way of dealing with long-buried issues.

Fear is a very natural emotion as we begin to lose weight. Many times, our biology, combined with our emotional reactivity, has been unable to handle one or more situations in our lives. Maybe we had a rough childhood, and took on issues that were not ours to take on. Maybe we were abused, or just had a sensitive nature. Adding weight is one common way we have of protecting themselves against these things we don't believe we can live up to.

So as you begin to take away this protective covering, fear usually makes an appearance. It's not as if we have to duplicate the exact situations we never dealt with before. But chances are, you may have other opportunities, in your contemporary life, to deal with similar issues. Your fear may manifest as bad dreams, troubled sleep, disturbing images in your mind, or even a trail of storylines in which you're the one being abandoned, rejected and subjected to failure.

Cultivating true emptiness here can help alleviate the natural inclination to exacerbate suffering, by limiting our attachment to the outcome of our actions. If we can learn to stop reacting to our stories, or lessen the emotional impact of this reactivity, we can achieve the kind of success we want to achieve. As well, we become the masters of our own lives, and can learn to define success for ourselves, taking into account our individual needs.

Meditation

This week's meditation will focus on how we tend to make our suffering worse, particularly as we try to take off excess weight. Our minds may play a starring role in this, so we'll delve into the ways your mind may be making things harder for you, perhaps without your permission. We'll also work on cultivating emptiness as a tool for weight loss, not just in terms of the sensation of being hungry or full, but as it relates to the various strong emotions that tend to come up whenever our protective covering has been removed.

Losing weight is, in a sense, losing part of yourself. The closer you get to learning who you are on a very intimate level, the more power you will have when emotional issues arise. None of us is perfect. We all have deep and varied histories. Using the tools of Meditation, Follow Up, Off the Mat Practice and Extending Your Practice with Story on a regular and sustained basis will help you reveal that history, and develop methods to cope with any difficulties that may arise.

Make sure to leave plenty of time after you meditate to record your experiences, memories and associations. Each nugget of information you uncover about yourself brings you one step closer to your ultimate goal.

- Go to your preferred meditation space, closing the door after you to ensure your privacy. If you don't have a door, try to pull a curtain, or do your meditation when no one else is around to distract you. Make sure you have your notebook and writing implement or mini-cassette recorder to record your experiences.

- Bring your body into your meditation posture, either seated on the floor, with your legs crossed, or in a chair, with your feet flat on the floor. Arrange the parts of your body so they form a solid foundation for your practice. Try to bring yourself upright, into a dignified position, but with a lightness that defies rigidity.

- When you've found a posture that feels balanced and supportive, move through the 7 Points of Posture in your mind, making tiny adjustments as you see fit. As a reminder, the 7 Points of Posture include: the seat and legs, the eyes and gaze, the spine, the shoulders, the neck and throat, the mouth and tongue, and the hands. Bring awareness to each part of your body as you further refine your posture.

- When you've finished bringing awareness to each part of your body, begin to connect each of your senses. Bring your attention to your eyes, your ears, your nose, your hands and your mouth, touching each one very lightly with your consciousness. Try to avoid making judgements about how each sense "should" be. Just notice how it is right now. Validate its contribution to your greater wellbeing.

- Now that you've made adjustments to your meditation posture and connected all of your senses to your practice, it's time to assume your Base Practice. Watch your breath as it moves in and out of your body, without trying to control the rate at which your body inhales or exhales. As you notice thoughts or storylines in your mind, say "thinking" to yourself and just let them ride your out breath.

- By now, you've been meditating for a few weeks, and you may have begun to notice your mind so well that you can "see" a thought before it carries you away. This is the inch of perspective that keeps us from reacting to challenging life situations, and deepening our suffering.

- Feel yourself in your body. Starting at the top and working down, take a look at all the parts of your body. Notice if one place is feeling tighter than another. Validate all you find, without trying to "correct" anything.

- When you feel ready to, bring forward an image of your own body. See it as if it's one of those models we all used in science class, where the body is transparent, and you can see all the internal organs inside. Make sure this body is yours, and has your face. Breathe in and out, feeling your body as a clear container, with your internal organs visible.

- Now see yourself as completely empty, without any organs at all. All of your veins and arteries are gone. All your fat and muscle tissues are gone. All of your skin is gone, along with the cartilage and bone that make up your skeleton. Breathe into this empty body, feeling the spaciousness inside yourself.

- Keep holding this image of yourself as empty and spacious as you see a bright green light illuminating you from inside. Keep breathing, keeping your concentration on the rising and falling of your chest, and the feeling of your breath in your mouth, your throat, and your lungs.

- When you look at yourself this way, how do you feel? What emotions are sparked as you feel the endless space inside you? Sit with any strong feelings that have come up in the meantime.

- Now do a quick glance through your body, this time starting from the bottom. How have your emotions changed the way you feel? Has tension lodged itself in any area that wasn't formerly feeling this way?

- As you sit with your feelings and the sensations in your body, notice the cartilage and bones coming back to inhabit your body, giving it structure. Notice your arteries and veins coming back to help the blood flow from place to place. And notice your internal organs coming back, fitting together in perfect harmony. Lastly, see your skin come back, to cover your body and protect it from harm. Take five full breaths here, staying with your body.

• Now focus on your head only. See your face from the front, smiling back at you. See yourself from the right side, the back side, and then the left side, as if your head were turning in a circle.

• Then, as you hold this image in mind, see your skin disappearing, your skull disappearing, your brain disappearing, your eyes, nasal passages, tongue and palate disappearing. See your blood vessels evaporate. All you're left with is true emptiness. This does not mean that you are "empty headed," or that you have nothing on your mind. It does not mean that your cares have disappeared. You know this already, because you can sense the endless, spacious nature of your own mind. Then see your mind filled with healing green light.

• Sit with this feeling of deep spaciousness as you check in with your emotions. How are you feeling now? Have any strong feelings come up for you at this time? Have you had any strong memories or associations?

• When you're finished checking in with your emotions, check in with the various parts of your body. Are you holding stress or tension anyplace new? Have certain places relaxed since the time you began this meditation? Just sit with whatever you find, knowing that whatever you find is exactly right for this moment.

• See all the parts of your head coming back to form you: the blood vessels and tongue, the palate and nasal passages. The eyes, brain and skull. See your skin coming back to cover your head. Return to your Base Practice, following your breath and labeling your thoughts when you notice them in your mind.

• Then come out of the meditation. Stay in your meditation posture for a few more seconds, maybe a minute or two, until you have your bearings again. Move slowly and deliberately as you return to your waking life.

Follow Up Exercise

As you come back into routine awareness, give yourself a few extra minutes. When you work with meditations involving strong visualizations like this last one, you may need a little more time to let your body and mind return to normal. Have patience with where you are right now. Get a glass of water, if you need to, and drink it very slowly.

When you feel ready, begin recording your experiences, using your notebook and writing implement or mini-cassette recorder. Remember to bypass your Internal Editor by being as authentic and real about your experiences as possible, even if they're unflattering.

Make sure to leave room for any thoughts, emotions or memories that do not have to do with the meditation, but which may have been freed as a result of doing it. If you've made an important association, such as your habit of overeating, and a memory of being afraid as you waited for your parents to come home from work, by all means follow the thread of that for a bit.

Start writing as soon as you feel ready, and try not to stop until you've said everything you want to say. As always, I'll include a few prompts here to get you started:

- Have you found a comfortable meditation posture for yourself?
- If so, how did you go about making adjustments?
- If not, how can you make adjustments in the next two weeks to support your practice?
- Were you able to run through the 7 Points of Posture with ease?
- How have you noticed your body changing over the past week?
- How have you noticed yourself present within your body during this time?
- Are you able to connect your senses to your meditation pretty easily?
- Has this had an effect on your senses in your waking life? If so, what kind of effect has it had?
- After you did this meditation, did you discover any old memories?
- If so, what were they, and how did they make you feel?

- Did you have any strong emotions come up during this meditation?
- If so, where did these emotions lodge themselves in your body?
- Were you able to see an image of yourself during the meditation?
- Could you see yourself as a transparent being?
- What did it feel like when you saw your organs and veins disappearing?
- What was the strongest emotion in you at that point in the meditation?
- Were you able to get in touch with the sense of being truly empty?
- How did you feel when you saw your body being filled with green light?
- When you began to focus on your head, were you able to visualize yourself easily?
- Did any strong feelings come up for you at this time?
- Did any strong sensations come up in your body?
- If so, where were they located?
- When you returned to your Base Practice, was it easier or harder than usual to watch your breathing and label your thoughts?
- Finally, as you closed your meditation, how were your feelings affected? Can you remember what the first thing in your mind was when you ended it?

Take your time. Let your innate creativity come forward as everything else recedes into the background. Know that you have personal storylines inside you, all the time, and that these storylines can help you form a clearer path toward your goals of losing weight and achieving your best body. Let yourself practice as if your hair were on fire, as some Buddhist teachers urge. Let that sense of urgency, to get at your innermost truths, take you over.

Please do the meditation and follow up exercise every day of the week (or so) you choose to practice with Emptiness. Let the concept of emptiness dissolve into you, rather than trying to understand it intellectually. New ways of looking at it may occur to you. Leave the door open to what you might find.

Off the Mat Practice

As you practice the meditation on Emptiness during this week, you're likely to have many opportunities to bring this practice off the mat and into your daily life. Keep noticing yourself in your body, at least once per day. Just as we practice meditation to tame the mind, or understand its workings and levels of reactivity, practicing with feeling yourself in your body at least once per day strengthens the concentration, and brings deeper understanding to your weight loss journey.

Emptiness, as we have seen, is often understood as the quantity of food in our stomachs, or the feeling we have when we haven't eaten much. But emptiness is also a very elevated aspect of enlightenment. Sages say it is the state during which humans perceive and understand all things to be impermanent. They know that happiness does not last, pain does not last, life does not last, and death does not last. They are also able to dispel any illusory thinking, such as the notion that we are separate from other people.

If we think about it, this has a direct application to weight loss. While we try to lose weight, we are all seeking, quite literally, to be enlightened. We want to feel lighter in our bodies. We want to be free of the metaphorical weight, of carrying too many emotional burdens. We want to be free of the emotional weight, of shame and anger and fear. And we also want to be free of the physical weight, which pulls us down to earth and endangers our overall health.

So as you take your practice off the mat and notice yourself in your body, take a moment right afterwards to feel the pull of gravity on your body, and then to release that mentally, allowing yourself to feel lighter and less burdened. Notice the feelings that come up for you as you do this, and any thoughts that run through your mind. Also notice any strong sensations in your body.

If you want to take it a step further, begin to notice the ways in which you get tripped up in expectations and outcomes. True emptiness is difficult to master because it means that we understand that, even as we strive to meet goals that may be very good for us in the long run, we may not be able to achieve what we want, or to achieve it within a certain prescribed time-frame.

Do you give up on diets a few weeks in because you haven't lost enough weight to justify giving up your favorite foods? Do you convince yourself that it's better to avoid exercising because the last time you tried it, it didn't achieve the outcome you'd hoped? Do you try to cut your caloric intake to dangerous levels because you need to speed up your weight loss?

For now, it's great if you can begin to see yourself thinking these types of thoughts, or engaging in these types of behaviors. There's no need to get caught up in whether they're "good" or "bad," or whether you need to do anything to change them. Bringing your awareness to their existence is already a huge step towards redirecting them in a healthy way.

Extend Your Practice with Story

Over the past seven weeks, you've added to a personal narrative of your own creation. Last week's addition included your thoughts and recollections about yourself as a child, and the time at which you first began to understand that you were different because of your size and shape. You talked about the early dynamics of your family, and how they factored into your own beliefs about yourself. Lastly, you wrote or spoke about the ways you've kept these family dynamics in place, or decided to leave them behind. If you left them behind, you also wrote a bit about why you had decided to do that.

Go back to the beginning of your personal narrative. Read it over in its entirety, taking your time and giving your words the validation they deserve. Allow yourself to get caught up in the writing, allowing yourself a smile when something is funny, or a wince when something is painful.

As always, resist the impulse to change anything, even if you notice a spelling mistake. It's not important that it be perfect; it's important that it be true. Then notice whether or not this personal narrative describes the way you feel today. Personal journeys that bring a great number of inner and outer change, such as weight loss, often bring quicksilver emotional changes. So there is no shame in feeling differently today. Just notice it and move on.

Find a fresh page in your notebook, or move to an unrecorded section of your mini-cassette tape. Spend a few moments calming your mind and focusing on your breath, just bringing yourself into the eternal present.

Then think about your life so far. Begin when you were a child, the parts of it you can remember, then moving into adolescence. Can you remember feeling as if you were nothing? Like no one could see you, or really appreciate who you were trying to be? Begin writing about how that situation played itself out in your life, including how it made you feel, what you did about it, and if there was ever a resolution.

Then move on into your teenage years and early adulthood. Try to find another time when you felt as if you were in danger of becoming non-existent, or completely invisible to others. Write another paragraph or two about that, making sure to remember as many details you can. Sights, smells, sounds and tactile sensations are wonderful ways to really cement the feeling for you, and to find a way of going even deeper into it. Include as many of them as you can.

If your Internal Editor makes an appearance, blow it off. Put your pen to the paper and keep writing. If you're speaking into a cassette recorder, just keep speaking, even if what you're saying sounds silly. You don't know when you will stumble on an important memory, or discover that you remember a lot more than you thought you did.

Finally, move into your adult years. You can choose a moment that happened last week, or one that took place years ago. Keep writing about how you experienced the sensation of being there and yet not being there. Where did this event take place? Who else was there? What did feeling empty make you want to do? Do you remember eating before or after this feeling? If so, what did the act of eating feel like at that time?

Now move on to a new paragraph. Explain how you may have contributed to any bad feelings by exacerbating them. Did your mind pile hurt on top of hurt? How so? Did you decide to hurt yourself before others could do it for you? Did that become a comfortable emotion for you to rest in, because it was so familiar?

Whatever you find, keep writing. Let everything spill out onto the paper—a description of the event or events, your feelings about them, your desires relative to the situation, and what you were left with after it was all done. Let your pen fly. Let your mind guide it along.

Now think about how your hopes were either fulfilled or dashed in these three separate instances. Did you extend yourself again and again, hoping to get what you secretly (or not so secretly) wanted? Or did you pull back into yourself, unwilling to risk being hurt? Were your hopes like wispy little ghosts, searching for someplace to land? If you were unable to bring your hopes to fruition, how did you gain ground, so you could feel stable and secure?

Let yourself open your mind from the inside. Try not to think about what you're writing. Try not to let your analytical faculties come into play. Instead, feel your sense of play awakened and your innate curiosity piqued as you explore the unknown terrain of your own psyche. Each inch you uncover should be filled with wonder and excitement.

Bring your awareness to a time in recent memory when you felt fear. It does not have to be the kind of fear you feel when you watch a horror movie. It doesn't have to feel as if you're being chased. Just think about the different kinds of fear you may feel on a day-to-day basis, such as fear of not making enough money, fear of old age and death, fear of being alone, fear of losing family members or loved ones, fear of not being accepted, or fear of accidents.

Then write about that moment, when you recall feeling the fear in you mind and in your body? How was your mind affected? Were you able to think clearly, or were you a bit clouded in your thinking? How was your body affected? Did your temperature rise, or seem to drop suddenly? Did you notice any particular sensations in your stomach? In your limbs or torso? In your head?

Keep writing, going into another paragraph or two if you need to. Fear is a very potent emotion when you are aware enough to notice it. Think about your recent attempts to lose weight and achieve your best body. Have you felt fear that you wouldn't be able to reach your goal? Worried, that your friends would treat you differently? Terrified, that people may not even recognize you for who you are?

At the end of this exercise, you may have 7-8 paragraphs, and perhaps more. Keep writing, if you need to. There's no set length for these exercises. They are meant to be prompts for you to look more deeply into yourself, and get to know your own mind a bit better. When you feel ready, put down your pen, or turn off your mini-cassette recorder.

Breathe. Center yourself. Then turn back (or rewind) to the beginning of what you wrote. Read everything you wrote today, reliving the three times you felt insubstantial or invisible in your life, the hopes you had that may or may not have been fulfilled, and the ways you tended to build ground under yourself for support. Lastly, listen to the fears that came up for you recently, and how they affected your mind and body. When you've finished reading over or listening to your work, put it aside for the week.

Know that you are free to return to your personal narrative at any time during the week, to add to it. You're not required to do this, though. Story is a practice, and the more you do it, the more comfortable you will feel. But telling your story needs to come naturally, or else you may begin to feel resentful.

Next week, we'll look at the concept of Enough. Establishing strong boundaries and understanding limits is one potent way of approaching the issue of extra weight in our lives. We'll look into all aspects of this crucial concept, including how to tolerate and accept the limits of our existence, and how to understand where the mind ends and the body begins. When we've had enough of our current situation, once and for all, there's nothing stopping us from changing. We merely need to understand where we are in our lives relative to where we want to be, then take action to embody the change we want to see. Taking that first step (or the 9th, 10th or 11th) may come directly from saying "enough," where we've met our edge and decided that to continue in the same direction would be fruitless.

Until then, have a great week, and don't forget to keep practicing!

Chapter Eight

> "The sheer size too, the excessive abundance, scale, and exaggeration of dreams could be an infantile characteristic. The most ardent wish of children is to grow up and get as big a share of everything as the grown-ups; they are hard to satisfy; do not know the meaning of 'enough.'"
>
> -- Sigmund Freud, *The Interpretation of Dreams*

Enough

You've made it through another week in this program—congratulations! Working with your mind and body together, as you've probably seen, has the effect of redoubling your efforts and clarifying your intentions, until they're far easier to enact. And as we learn how our minds can shape our reality, by determining what we see or don't see around us, we strengthen our resolve and our skill at getting what we want.

This week, we'll practice with the concept of Enough. No doubt you'll have a series of mental and emotional reactions of your own when you hear that word. But in delving into our limits, as beings incarnate in human bodies, we can see how our boundaries may need strengthening during a program of weight loss, in order to see where we end, literally and figuratively, and where others begin.

But first, let's take a moment to check in from last week:

- Did you do your meditation exercises every day of the week (or more) you decided to practice with Emptiness?
- How did you find your daily meditation sessions?
- Did you look forward to them, or dread doing them every day?
- Have you noticed a willingness to make more time for yourself?
- If not, have you gotten more adept at identifying any obstacles that still stand in your way?
- How do you find your meditation posture these days?

- Have you been able to steadily tweak your meditation posture so that you can sit on the cushion more upright and dignified, but without tension or undue pain?
- Have you been able to run through the 7 Points of Posture, without having to be reminded of each one?
- If not, what steps might you take in order to bring this awareness to your practice?
- As you bring more balance to your meditation posture, have you found that you feel more balanced in your life?
- How are you doing in connecting your senses to your meditation?
- Has any one sense seemed to awaken more than the others?
- Has your sensory experience of your daily life also been awakened, to some degree?
- What new information have you been able to gather about your world?
- Do you remember having any strong feelings before you began the visualization part of the meditation?
- If so, what were they?
- Were your feelings consistent from day to day?
- When you saw your body as a collection of organs and arteries, how did you feel?
- Were you able to get in touch with the feeling of spaciousness?
- Were any of your feelings concentrated in any one part of your body?
- How did it feel to see your body as empty of skin or contents?
- Were you able to send healing green light into your body?
- How did that feel?
- Did you see your head as a skull, brain and related material?
- How did it feel to see your mind as truly and literally empty?
- Were you able to fill your head with healing green light as well?
- Did you make sure to leave yourself plenty of time to record your experiences during the Follow Up Exercise?
- In your Off the Mat Practice, were you able to keep feeling yourself in your body, at least once per day?
- Were you able to get in touch with the feeling of gravity, and practice allowing yourself to feel more enlightened when you mentally released it?

- Were you able to identify instances when you tend to get caught up in outcomes and expectations?
- If so, what were they?
- When you identified these instances, did any strong feelings come up for you?
- Were you able to simply identify them, without trying to make them "better"?
- When you did the Extend Your Practice with Story exercise, were you able to remember two instances when you felt small, invisible or "less than"?
- How were your feelings affected by remembering this sense of being non-existent?
- Were you able to add details such as textures, colors, smells and sounds to your personal narrative?
- Did you see how your mind may have exacerbated the pain of that time for you?
- How were your hopes and desires fulfilled or dashed in these instances?
- How did you attempt to bring more grounding to your situation?
- Were you able to bring forward a memory of fear?
- Did you notice where your fear tends to gather in your body?
- Are any of your fears related to your body, or the journey of losing weight?
- Finally, how are you feeling right now about your body?

The same rules apply here as when you Extend Your Practice with Story. Let your pen fly over the page, so fast that your Internal Editor can't keep up. When you've finished with the prompt questions above, try looking into yourself exactly as you are now, and write about that. It doesn't matter if it sounds silly. It doesn't mater if it's not earth-shattering prose. What's important is that you employ the tools you have at hand to understand your mind, and how it contributes to any problems you may be trying to solve.

When you're finished writing or speaking your truth, sit with whatever feelings, thoughts or bodily sensations you have at this moment. Maybe the feeling doesn't have a name. Try to name it, even if you call it Harry or Teapot or Postage Stamp. Maybe your feelings are a combination of several individual emotions. Write it down or speak it into your recorder. This is your time, your mind, and your body. Treat them all, even if just for this moment, as if they're the most important things on earth.

The Limits of our Existence

The *American Heritage Dictionary* defines *enough* as "sufficient to meet a need or satisfy a desire; adequate." It is an adjective, a pronoun, an adverb and an interjection. The word derives from Indo-European roots, meaning "to get," or "to carry," and has developed into our current usage through Old and Middle English.

In our contemporary usage, the word *enough* implies all kinds of limits on our existence. We make sure our dish is cooked enough, but not too much. We are happy enough with the raise we got at work. We've had enough when someone irritates us. We may even express our exasperation by saying, "Enough!"

Like *weight*, this is a word that carries many implications in our language. Similarly, it also expresses the places where we come up against the edge of our patience, our good will, or our endurance. Because of this, it's a concept that applies very directly to the act of losing weight and trying to achieve our best bodies.

Our culture is saturated with negative messages about carrying too much weight—that much is obvious. But where does our personal sovereignty end and that of others begin? When are we securing our overall health, and when are we devolving into narcissism and unhealthy, self-punishing behaviors? And what about the line of demarcation between our minds and bodies, or between our minds, bodies and souls?

To answer these questions, we must get more deeply in touch with the concept of *enough*, and how it applies to the individual circumstances of our lives.

Understanding Our Own Limits

One of the reasons we are so image-obsessed as a culture is because we need to project our realities in some way. We've invented photographs, movies and television as safe places to visit when we're not feeling so great about our lives. We can usually find a character to identify with, and then project ourselves into their skin. We identify so much that, by the end of some shows, we're crying along with the protagonists.

Even the most coolly bored among us aren't immune from this experience. It's as if our nightly dreams have come alive in living color, for all to see. Photographs, movies and television can also achieve important social changes in a fraction of the time it would take without them. Because of photography, we can learn about cultures across the globe, in places so remote we may never have the chance to visit them otherwise. Movies have made it possible to "live" in a computer-generated world. And television has increasingly led to greater acceptance of formerly marginalized groups like blacks, gays, Latinos and women.

In these contained worlds, the only limits are those of the time-slot the show occupies. That may be one reason we're drawn to them. But in our real lives, we have all kinds of limits that we experience every day. We can't be everywhere. We can't do everything. We can't control the outcome of many events. But the fact of limitation is the reason we can also experience transformative emotions like compassion.

Most people understand having compassion to mean being nice to someone. It can range from the kind of "nice" that more closely resembles pity, where someone is seeing themselves as separate from or better than someone else. Or it can become a benign form of behaving in a pleasant manner, which ruffles no feathers and causes no waves.

But the story told most frequently to demonstrate what compassion really means is that of an armless mother whose baby has fallen into a river. Terrified, the mother races along the muddy banks, trying to save her child. But she has no way to reach out, and the current is swift. In a flash, it carries the baby away.

This could be read as a dire warning to mothers, to never let their children out of their sight. It could make you feel terribly sad, that a tiny, defenseless creature had to die. And all of those are part of the feeling behind compassion. We want the best for others and ourselves, and want to cause no harm. We ache with our inability to effect change. But circumstances are often beyond our control. And sometimes, there's nothing at all we can do but watch, with our feelings deeply pained, as someone or something is whisked from our grasp.

149

Applying compassion to ourselves as part of a plan to eat healthier foods, lose weight and exercise demands that we understand where the limits of our existence lie. We cannot assume that we will be a size 4 when everyone in our family wears at least a 12. We can't kill ourselves with unhealthy mental and physical patterns while trying to "save" ourselves from obesity. And ultimately, it probably won't matter what size we are when we die. The point is to raise those pained feelings of compassion for yourself, as if you were that terrified mother on the banks of the river, watching something you loved be carried away. What can you do about the situation you find yourself in now? And what is completely and irrevocably beyond your control?

Where the Mind Ends and the Body Begins

About a year ago, I was working with a client who wanted to write a memoir about his early years. His mother, a kind and widely admired local woman, had wanted a girl when he was born, so she continued to dress him in girl's clothing for much of his young life. As any child would, he relished the attention he received from his mother, and went along with her preferences without thinking twice. But as he grew older and began to attend school, Kyle (not his real name) came up against the standard conditioning most of us go through according to our gender.

Kyle had a rough time, not just because he was teased about the clothing he wore, and the decidedly feminine way he held and expressed himself. His crisis also included having to make the terrible choice between his cherished relationship with his mother, whom he was hesitant to challenge, and his own self, which had to go to school every day to cruel taunts.

At the same time, Kyle began to gain weight. His mother wasn't the facilitator of this weight gain, but she didn't exactly dissuade him from eating more than three meals a day, and lavish snacks when he returned home from school. Food was one way they bonded, along with cooking at mealtimes and holidays.

For a time, Kyle struggled with his conundrum. Did he enjoy dressing in girls' clothing because he liked it, or was it to please his mother? Was he gay, like some of the other children suggested? Where, precisely, did his mother end and he begin?

People who tend to carry added weight often struggle with these sorts of dilemmas. You don't have to have a mother who dressed you in clothing opposite to your gender, or have even experienced terrible parenting of any sort. As I've mentioned before, every infant has a thousand ways to detect what's "correct" and what's not, what's socially acceptable and what can't be tolerated. We don't need someone yelling, or writing a giant message on a billboard to understand that, on some deep level, we've crossed a line by not adhering to the size constraints placed on us.

This is where the mind ends and the body begins. Our thoughts about ourselves may be accepting and tolerant. This is the reality of our minds. But when we're placed in the larger social environment of our schools, our jobs, and our communities, what we believe about ourselves is tested again and again. People tell us we're fat. They shun us or try to make us feel unwelcome. This is the reality of our bodies.

In order to bridge the gap between mind and body, we have to make a choice. We can choose to go with what our minds tell us is the truth, that we're good people, no matter what the number on the scale says. We can choose to believe the outside world, which may tell us that to be overweight is to doom ourselves to a lifetime of loneliness. Or maybe the answer lies somewhere in between.

Ultimately, Kyle chose himself, ultimately asking his mother to take him to Sears for some clothing more suited to a young boy. Silently, his mother obliged him, but their relationship was never the same. As he and I worked together to unearth some of his most potent memories, I asked if he'd ever stopped loving his mother, or blamed her for what had happened. But all Kyle could remember was how fiercely he loved her, and how he knew that she felt the same away about him.

When Kyle's mother died in 1999, it took him six months to stop grieving openly. When he saw little girls running for their school bus, he broke down crying. When he went to the mall to try on clothing, his hands shook. It took Kyle several years in therapy to work on the separation between himself and his mother that should have taken place as a normal part of maturation process. But there was still the issue of his mind and memories, and how they related to his body.

In our work together, Kyle and I focused on re-establishing the limits of his existence. He had never really tested himself against what he found comfortable, since he was always living for what he believed his mother wanted from him. So at 45, Kyle began to experience where his edges were, physically, emotionally, mentally and spiritually.

Some of us need huge transformative events like a parent dying in order to realize that it's time to change. Our days become so filled with the events we call "living" that we forget that we have boundaries, or that our limits sometimes need to be defined, redefined and strengthened, especially if we're thinking about changing the food we eat and the way we burn calories. More on this in a minute.

Other times, may just come to the end of our emotional rope. We may be sick of looking at a body that just doesn't feel like us anymore, or feel lonely when we don't have the companionship we desire. We may even desire to do things our current bodies will not allow us to do, and struggle against our limitations.

There are many positive reasons to change the size or shape of one's body, including generalized health reasons, such as congenital heart problems, or risks of diabetes and cancer. You may want to feel more present in yourself, or assist the development of your mind-body connection. You may even want to change your eating patterns to deal with allergies and digestive problems caused by the foods you're currently eating.

However, there are probably just as many negative reasons to change the size and shape of your body, and many of them can result in increased health problems, many of which mirror the ones we may be trying to get away from … like heart disease, diabetes and cancer, among others. Trying to become as small as possible may not end up making you happier, even though it may seem that way when you're not where you want to be. But attempting to wear a particular size to compete with others, or show up someone you don't like may only end up causing you to feel as small as your waistline is becoming.

The point is that there's no one body type that's right for everyone, just as there is no right weight or size. I don't even like to use the word *diet*, because it often comes with horrible associations of deprivation and hunger. Instead, I like to think of food as a source of medicine. When I eat well, meaning I get balanced sources of fruit, grains, vegetables and protein, I feel as if I'm taking the medicine that will make my body run correctly. When I don't, I can feel the effects of what I've taken into my body almost immediately.

Achieving your best body means finding the combination of size, shape, food and exercise that's right for you, your genes, your lifestyle and your goals. That means no one else, not that model on the cover of the magazine, not that "helpful" spouse, and not that hectoring parent, should come into it. It's all you from here on out.

Establishing Stronger Boundaries

In this day and age, everyone who's tried to make a life change has probably read at least one self-help book. And that means you may have become familiar with the concept of personal boundaries as they relate to our relationships and working lives. But few, if any, people talk about boundaries as regards our bodies during the process of losing weight.

Our boundaries, for those who may not have any experience with this concept, are where we end and public space begins. This may be an invisible line that separates our "personal space" from that of others. And we all know how uncomfortable it can be if someone, knowingly or unknowingly, violates this invisible line. It can be an invisible emotional line that we just don't cross with other people. For instance, most people don't draw attention to the fact that we're looking a little heavier, just as we don't point out that we know their wife has been cheating on them for the past six months.

This invisible line may also extend to our minds, forming a place we will allow ourselves to go (fantasizing about a wonderful vacation in Tahiti, for example), along with places we will not allow ourselves to go (what happens if I remain overweight and no one decides to love me?). In these two examples, our mind is a separate entity, either helping us get through a challenging work situation by allowing us to picture what it'll be like when we're lying on the beach, or causing us to rub salt in our emotional wounds.

As we've seen so far in this program, meditation is a tool that can help us become more familiar with how our minds work. It can help us determine whether our minds are providing that helpful, encouraging voice in the back of our minds, or creating a horror show of terrifying images intent on keeping us from achieving whatever's healthiest for us.

If you've experienced more of the latter in your meditations so far, it may be time to strengthen your boundaries. These begin on the inside, and can then be built up and extended into the outside world. If we know how we feel when someone gets too close too soon, either on an emotional or physical level, we may feel the need to reinforce this boundary with food. Weight, after all, can keep people away more effectively than practically any other means.

If you find that you've inadvertently been keeping people away with your weight (we'll explore this a little more in this week's meditation), as a kind of external boundary, there's no reason to berate yourself or feel ashamed. There is a reason your emotional support system may have needed this distance. Delving deeper to find the reasons for your discomfort may provide crucial insight that can help you take off the weight once and for all, and relax into a life of greater intimacy. In the next few sections, we'll work on how to recognize and most importantly, determine for yourself if you need to strengthen or relax your boundaries.

Getting to Enough (and Staying There)

When someone comes too close for comfort, or invades our boundaries in some way, we grow uncomfortable. We may not even use the word *boundaries*, but we know that bad feeling of having been transgressed somehow. We may react quickly and violently, telling someone in no uncertain terms to back off, or we may let it fester inside us, not understanding why we feel this way, and therefore not understanding what to do about it.

There's no such thing as a correct or incorrect response when it comes to feeling transgressed. The bottom line is that someone or some situation has pressed us against our edge, the limit of what we can take on a mental or emotional level. We may be aware of that edge, or completely, blissfully unaware of it. But I believe we encounter troublesome people and these irritating situations when we need to find where our edge is, and most likely do something about it. Losing weight is one of those journeys in life that tend to bring in a lot of this sort of energy.

It may be because adding weight to your body, whether it's intentional, unintentional, genetic, caused by illness or medication, or even from sheer laziness, fosters a kind of forgetting. When we add more weight than our bodies need to feed our organs and support our bones, we add layers of fat and skin over whatever's already there—feelings, mental associations, self-beliefs and other energetic patterns. Having the extra weight there sometimes makes it hard to contact these original feelings. And because our feelings are farther away, our responses to them are far away as well. They take longer to realize, and longer to react to. They may lie dormant or buried in that state for years.

This may contribute to not even realizing that your boundaries are being ignored, or that you're having certain feelings because that's what's happening in your life. It may be at the root of your unhappy feelings about your weight, but not realizing that it's far more than cosmetic changes you want to make. It is my strong belief that diets simply don't work. Periods of starvation followed by eating whatever you missed out on only has the effect of sending your weight fluctuating in a way that's dangerous for your health. The key to losing weight lies in locating your edge, becoming very comfortable with it, and then vowing to protect it no matter what.

When someone moves across our emotional or personal space boundaries without our permission, we say, "Enough!" Whether it's verbal or non-verbal, we know that we've met our edge, determined that we cannot be moved any further beyond it, and made up our minds to stop whatever force is trying to encroach on our emotions. The same is true for losing weight and achieving your best body.

Each of us must be vigilant about our boundaries—the mental, spiritual, emotional and physical. If we don't know what makes us uncomfortable now, we must become increasingly aware of what does, and in what types of situations. Meditation can help you develop this deeper personal awareness. The Follow Up Exercises can help you venture a little deeper into these uncharted territories, and help you take risks in small, controlled ways. Extending Your Practice with Story can help bring these moments of discomfort alive in a way that will be hard for you to forget.

When you begin to value yourself in this way, your self-esteem will improve. You don't have to lose weight in order to do this. In fact, I've found that the process works better the other way around. Increasing your level of self-esteem will help you realize that every living person has the right to dignity, and being treated with respect. You will find that you are one of those lucky people, and that getting to enough, and staying there, may not be as difficult as it seems.

Meditation

In this week's meditation, we'll spend some time looking at our "edge," and how coming up against it gives us a choice, right in that moment, to do something positive for ourselves, or to do something with neutral or potentially negative effects. As usual, our minds play a key role in deciding how our bodies will react, and we'll look into why mental decisions sometimes help to keep weight on, or help it come off faster.

It may be easier said than done to say, "Enough," and push away from the table. This is oversimplifying the problem of added weight. Of course, if we put more food into our bodies, more than it needs for us to function, the more we are apt to weigh. But just as thousands of tiny functions band together to help us create a song, or walk to the store, or bake a cake, thousands of ideas, beliefs and thoughts can combine to facilitate weight loss, or to leave things exactly as they are now.

This week's meditation addresses the needs inside all of us to be safe and nurtured, and can help you to see where you may need more of that energy in your life.

- Make your way to your meditation space, and close the door for privacy. It's important to make sure there are as few distractions as possible, so please try to choose the time and place of your meditations wisely. Don't forget to bring your notebook and a writing implement, so you can record your experiences later.

- Arrange your body into your meditation posture. Seat yourself on the floor, on a mat, or on a cushion, with your legs crossed under you. Or, if you have back or leg issues that prevent you from being able to sit this way, seat yourself in a chair, and place your feet flat on the floor. Inhale deeply, and bring yourself into an upright and dignified position as you exhale.

- As you bring your body into your meditation posture, mentally go through the 7 Points of Posture. If you need to, make tiny adjustments to your posture so it completely supports your weight. In case you need a reminder, the 7 Points of Posture include: the seat and legs, the eyes and gaze, the spine, the shoulders, the neck and throat, the mouth and tongue, and the hands.

- When you feel ready, connect each of your senses to your meditation. Bring your attention to your eyes and say "seeing" to yourself. Bring your attention to your ears and say "hearing" to yourself. Bring your attention to your nose and say "smelling" to yourself. Bring your attention to your mouth and say "tasting" to yourself. And lastly, bring your attention to your hands and say "touching" to yourself.

- Start your Base Practice, watching your breath as it moves in and out of your body, and labeling your thoughts as you notice them in your mind by saying "thinking" to yourself.

- As you notice thoughts or storylines in your mind, take note of the quality of the thoughts. For example, are you focused on something that happened today, perhaps an argument or missed opportunity? Are you focused on the future, such as what you'll have for dinner tonight, or how you'll confront a friend tomorrow? Or are your thoughts somewhere in the middle?

- When you have a pretty good sense about where you are mentally right now, take a quick look through the parts of your body, noticing where anything is tense or loose, where any part feels different than normal. Also take a moment to notice what it feels like to be in your body, since so many times, we're not used to doing that.

- Now bring forward a time when you felt that someone came too close for your comfort. It may be a friend who stepped inside the bubble of "personal space" we all have. It could be a boss who said something inappropriate to you at work. Or it may be someone who had the best intentions, but simply pushed us further and faster than we were comfortable going. Maybe you were the one who tried to push someone past his or her comfort zone.

- When you have this moment in mind, let it rest there. See yourself on the giving or receiving end of whatever was said or done. See yourself reacting as you reacted, and then feeling the feelings you felt. Get in touch with what the feelings are, as well as where they're resting in your body.

- Right at the moment when the line was crossed, try to "freeze the film" in your mind. Rather than letting the scene play out as it did in real life, let that moment remain stagnant. Then draw an imaginary line, or build an imaginary wall between you and this other person, right at the place where your comfort zone was diminished.

- This is where your boundaries were, even if you didn't know it at the time. Your boundary may be physical, such as the personal space barrier, or it may be emotional. Maybe someone pushed you further than you were ready to go in a relationship, or maybe someone showed you no respect when they asked you to perform a task without regard to your safety.

- For now, just sit with this boundary for a few breaths. Let the oxygen move through your lungs as you deepen your understanding of this "edge" we all have.

- When you feel ready, go back to the image in your mind—the "frozen" picture of your uncomfortable situation. See you, the other person, and this invisible line or wall you've constructed between. Go back and erase that line, or knock down that wall. In its place, draw another line, or build another wall that's about two feet closer to the person you're interacting with. This is where your edge is, the spot where most of us would prefer to stop, before our "line" is crossed.

- As before, just sit with this new image of yourself with a new, more comfortable boundary. If the issue is emotional rather than physical, see the place right before the other person made you uncomfortable. Move the line back accordingly.

- Keep breathing. Let your chest rise and fall like the waves of the ocean. Check in with the various parts of your body, to see if anything has changed during your meditation.

- Let the image in your mind go and return to your Base Practice. Take five full breaths here, labeling your thoughts by saying "thinking" to yourself. Let the thoughts dissipate on your out breath.

- Come out of the meditation. Give yourself plenty of time to come back to waking consciousness. Take your time rising from the mat, and returning to the normal business of your day.

Follow Up Exercise

After you've given yourself a few moments to get a glass of water or move around, come back to your meditation space to record your experiences. Get out your notebook, turn to a fresh page and begin writing off the top of your head, or use your mini-cassette recorder to record your experiences. Remember that sometimes, your thoughts may not make sense. They may not seem to relate to the meditation you've just done, or to the subject of this chapter. But watching your mind in meditation can have all kinds of unexpected results. That's why it's crucial to record all of your experiences, even if you feel they're weird, unrelated, embarrassing, etc. That may be where the real "meat" of the problems lies.

Let your pen fly as you remember the emotions that arose in you during this meditation session. Let it remember your physical sensations, especially if they seemed to be linked to any emotional fluctuations. And allow the act of writing to free you of any desire to clamp down on yourself, whether it's for what you ate today, what you wanted to eat, or what you may look alike at this moment. None of it matters. None of it is relevant to the stories trying to get out of you.

Here are a few prompts to get you started:

- During this meditation, how did you find your meditation posture?
- Do you allow yourself to make adjustments to your posture, or do you stick with it, even though it causes your body pain?
- How do you find working with the 7 Points of Posture these days?

- Have you noticed a shift in the relationship between your mind and body?
- If so, how would you describe this shift?
- How do you find working with your senses? Are they easy or hard for you to access?
- Do you find your senses more awakened as a result of doing these practices?
- Were any memories dislodged as a result of doing this meditation?
- If so, what were they?
- How were your emotions affected by doing this meditation?
- How was your body affected by doing this meditation?
- Were you able to remember a time in recent memory in which someone came too close for comfort?
- Were you the person crossing the line, or was your line crossed when this happened?
- Did you notice how your personal space was invaded?
- Were you able to see how you reacted to this moment?
- Were you able to get in touch with the feelings you had?
- Were you able to "freeze the film" in your mind, and imagine a line drawn between you and this other person?
- How did it feel to see where your boundary lay?
- Were you able to draw another line, further away, which increased your comfort zone?
- How did it feel to sit with that more comfortable "edge," or boundary?
- How was your body affected by moving this line?
- How were your emotions affected?
- When you came out of the meditation, what were you left with, mentally, emotionally, physically and spiritually?

While you're letting your pen take down everything your mind has to offer you now, the impulse may be to rush through it, or somehow get the writing aspect of this out of the way, like a chore. But this is the key component of this practice, and the one I've found from firsthand experience delineates what works from what doesn't. Take the time to get to know yourself. You may be surprised that when you do, others will as well.

For each day of the week that passes during the week or more you choose to practice with Enough, please remember to do your meditation exercises, preferably for a period of 10-20 minutes each. If you have more time, by all means practice for longer periods of time. But even if you're the most time-strapped person on the planet, please try to find at least ten minutes to increase your level of intimacy with yourself. Achieving your best body may depend on it.

Off the Mat Practice

Enough is a loaded concept for many people struggling with the concept of weight, with how much and how often to eat, and with what role food really plays in their lives. As well, practicing with Enough may reveal additional issues related to the hidden reasons we carry extra weight when our bodies don't seem to need it. For this week, begin by bringing more awareness to those instances in which your life presses us up against your edges.

This may mean that you notice your mind hardening against someone who always asks you to do things for them, even if that person hasn't said a word to you all week. It may mean owning the fact that you allowed someone to walk all over your feelings, just so *their* feelings were not hurt in any way. Or it may mean revealing to yourself that when people get too close to you, by invading your personal space, you suffer adverse physical or emotional effects.

Discovering moments when we feel terribly raw is not meant to be an exercise in self-torture. Instead, it's meant to help you bring greater awareness to the small interactions that make up our days. It's in these small moments when we allow ourselves to come up against our boundaries, stop short of them, or move wildly beyond them, so our lives are filled with a kind of permanent discomfort.

I have found, in years of working with my own life and with the lives of my clients, that heavy people tend to fall into the latter camp. Because of their early training, or subsequent choices they've made for themselves, these people tend to allow others to transgress their boundaries, or not even be aware of their boundaries. Adding weight then becomes a way of enforcing boundaries with sheer girth. If we can't get people to stay a respectful distance from us, we'll simply make it impossible for them to get any closer.

As you discover your boundaries this week, think about how you might also want to shift them. Sometimes, out of guilt of societal pressure, we adjust where our boundaries would naturally fall because we don't want to seem "high maintenance" or "diva-esque." Bringing some added attention to where you actually feel comfortable, and then suddenly don't, requires some fine-tuning. This can only happen if you take each small moment of your life at a time, testing out how each way of behaving feels, and then making adjustments as necessary.

Remember to feel yourself in your body at least once per day, both while still, either lying down or standing, and then moving through space in some way. Feel yourself being pulled toward the core of the earth by gravity, and then immediately release that feeling so you also experience how it feels to be weightless and light.

Finally, try to take your Off the Mat Practice a bit further, even if you do this just once during the week. After you're more comfortable noticing your edge, try to notice it a little earlier each time. Try seeing if you're going to feel uncomfortable within ten seconds, or two seconds, or a minute. Begin to notice how your body reacts when it knows it's being herded toward its edge. See how your mind reacts, and also how your emotions are stirred up in these moments.

If you can, try to pick one moment of each day. Say "enough" to yourself and stop yourself in your tracks. Right there. This could mean saying "enough" when it comes to eating, and stopping yourself a few bites short of being full. It could mean saying "enough" to yourself and keeping yourself from saying or doing something that might encourage someone (inadvertently) to transgress your boundaries. Or it could also mean saying "enough" in the midst of an unproductive or even self-destructive thought or storyline that enters your mind.

If you can think of other ways to take your practice off the mat, try them out. There is no harm in doing a little safe experimenting, to see how it feels to adjust where your boundaries are, and how it feels to let others know they're there. If you have emotional reactions or "little voices" that come up in response to these experiments, notice these as well. No need to do anything to change them at this point. The inner work you're doing each week, as long as it's done consistently, will shift your perspective over time.

Extend Your Practice with Story

Eight weeks ago, you began a personal narrative that described your reality at that point in time. Over these past few weeks, you've slowly been adding to it as we moved through the meditations and exercises in this book. Last week, your focus was on non-existence, and being over-looked or emotionally abandoned because of your size. You may have had thoughts or memories related to your visibility as a human being, as well as the feelings that accompanied those circumstances.

Before we begin this week, I want you to go all the way back to the beginning of your personal narrative. Read it over from start to finish, taking as long as you need to give your words the respect they deserve. If you find yourself getting caught up in the writing, let yourself be swept away emotionally. Experience everything again, if that's what you need to do.

Remember, there's no editing now, even if you find a spelling mistake. That was your reality on those days, and it's just as valid today as it was then. If you feel really different from the person you were when you wrote some of those words, good for you. That means the inner work you're doing is already having a profound effect.

Then go to a fresh page in your notebook and take the entry at the top. If you're using a mini-cassette recorder, go to an unrecorded section of tape, or change the tape if necessary. Center yourself by bringing your attention inward, and even concentrating on your breath for a few moments, if that helps you establish your focus.

Then think about your early life. Go back as far as you can remember right now, to a time when you felt your limits were not respected. This can be as simple as having an opinion at the age of two, and not having anyone listen. Or it could be a lot more complex, such as physical or even sexual abuse. How did having your limits ignored or transgressed make your dreams fade into the background? How did they contribute to the division between your body and mind?

Before you have a chance to think about it too much, or allow your Internal Editor into the room, begin to write or speak. It doesn't matter if what you have to say isn't perfectly edited, or well thought out. It doesn't matter if you stammer into the mini-cassette recorder, or stop frequently to collect your thoughts. Just think about one or more times in your early life when you felt overlooked, ignored, or aggressively shunted to the side.

Keep writing as you move into your adolescent years. Think of another instance when your limits came into play. Were they physical or emotional boundaries? How did you meet your edge? Were you even aware that it was there all along? Try to be as specific as you can as you allow your mind to free associate around this topic. If all you can come up with is a series of brief words and phrases describing your emotional reactions, that's fine, too. Try to get to the place where you feel completely free just letting it all come forward.

If you have additional memories, write about them as well. Include the smallest details you can remember, even if you feel they're not important to your personal narrative. As you move into your adult years, and remember one final time when you felt yourself coming up against your limits, get even deeper into the situation as you remember it. What did it smell like, taste like, sound like? What were the dominant colors and textures? What were you touching at the time, or wanting to touch? Finally, how was your body affected as you experienced this situation?

Start a new paragraph. Think about how your limits may have become either completely invisible to you as a result of simply forgetting, or very present for you, because your life was made uncomfortable by their existence. Do not hold back as you hold your emotional life to the light. Do not allow yourself to get into blaming others for your feelings, or somehow wanting to go back and do it over again. Just keep writing, remembering to include any times you added to your own hurt and confusion by judging yourself, or the feelings you were having.

When you've finished with that, add another paragraph or two on the dreams you've had over the course of your life. They may be very strong dreams, which have persevered for many years, or smaller dreams you've had only recently, and may be afraid to admit to yourself. Whatever pops to mind first, go with it.

Think about this dream. Get it down as accurately as you can on paper, or on your tape. Then think about how you went after your dreams, or allowed your limits to determine whether or not you reached for them. If you're in the latter camp, write down any and all limits you feel were placed on you, whether they were mental, emotional, physical, spiritual or financial in nature.

If your mind strays back to the writing itself, in an intellectual way, stop yourself right there. Push aside anything that wants to get in your way and make your only thought the freedom of writing or speaking into your recorder. Begin to associate this act of Extending Your Practice with Story with release, when nothing you say is wrong, and nothing you think or remember can have an adverse effect on anyone.

How did you identify your dream? What especially open part of yourself wanted to do that, and why? Try to get in touch with all the reasons you wanted to release any limits placed on you, so you could live on, and do this one thing. What makes you identify with this dream? What part of you responds most fervently when you think about doing it, or having it?

Keep moving, adding another paragraph about how your dreams have been subverted or shoved aside in this lifetime (if they have). Why have you not had the chance to meet your dreams? Have you given up on them entirely? Replaced them with new dreams? Or continued to chase them the best you know how?

How would it feel to have no physical limitations? How would it feel to be able to release the fear that sometimes contributes to mental or emotional fears, which hold all of us back? Write on, as you explore the physical and emotional responses you have when you think about releasing all the limits on your mind, your body and all the cells of your body, which hold your emotions.

By the end of this exercise, you may have 8-10 paragraphs, depending on how many new memories came up for you. If you need to, keep writing past this point, or stop short of it, if you've said all you need to say. When you're ready to do so, turn off your mini-cassette recorder or stop writing, and put your pen down.

Take a few moments to center yourself again, and go back to the beginning of what you wrote or spoke. Read everything over, standing in witness to what you've just uncovered about yourself. Let yourself realize, perhaps for the first time, how important our "edge" is, and how it serves to facilitate or limit our ability to think about ourselves in an active and healthy way.

When you've finished reading over your work, put it aside for now. If you feel you want to, please feel free to return to your personal narrative during the week. Begin to think of building your personal narrative as a practice, which needs to become second nature to you, like brushing your teeth or taking a shower. In time, your stories will flow out of you readily.

Next week begins the last week of our program towards achieving our best bodies. We'll work with the ways we can all bring ourselves out of our heads and down to earth. As we have seen, added weight has a way of bringing us in touch with earthly energies, sometimes literally. Allowing ourselves to return to the earth whenever we need to without eating too much, or allowing our energies to stagnate, can help us find our best bodies not just in the physical sense, but in the emotional, mental and spiritual senses as well.

Until then, please remember to practice every day, both with your mind, in meditation, and with your body, using the Follow Up and Off the Mat Exercises in this chapter. I believe that with sustained and devoted practice, you will find yourself not only clearing away old, negative self-beliefs, but forming the foundation of new beliefs, that you can make startling changes to your body, in concrete and healthful ways.

Chapter Nine

> "This outward spring and garden are
> a reflection of the inward garden."
>
> -- Mevlana Jelalu'ddin Rumi

Down to Earth

This is the ninth and final week of our program together, and I want to begin by thanking you for accompanying me on this journey. Deciding to engage with your mind-body connection is never an easy one, despite the plethora of self-help books out there. And taking the sustained action required to dig out old ways of being that no longer serve you is a brave act that few can claim.

With that being said, we'll work on coming back Down to Earth this week. In chapter 2, I talked about the connection between added weight and the element of earth. Some of those words may have seemed resonant to your individual relationships with your body and your weight. But this week, we'll explore ways to connect with that earthy energy without eating more than we need, or adding weight we may not feel like having on our frames.

But first, let's take a moment to check in from last week:

- In the time you decided to practice with Enough, did you get to do your meditation exercises every day?
- Did your meditation sessions have anything in common, such as an overriding emotional current, or mental pattern?
- How do you react emotionally when you think about doing your meditation exercises these days? Does it seem like a comfort, or a chore, or both?

- How has your life changed when it comes to establishing "your" time, as separate from the time you afford to other people and activities in your life?
- Have you implemented strategies for overcoming any obstacles that still stand in your way?
- If so, what do they entail?
- Are you happy with the meditation posture you've adopted?
- Are you able to sit in meditation for 20 to 30 minutes at a time, without experiencing pain or undue discomfort?
- Are you able to remember the 7 Points of Posture each time you meditate?
- If not, how can you go about reminding yourself?
- When you connect your senses to the meditation, how do you feel?
- Has any one sense seemed more "awake" than another?
- If so, which one? And why do you think that might be?
- Have you noticed any changes in your day-to-day reality, as a result of this practice?
- When you visualized a recent time when someone came too close for comfort, how did you feel?
- Did you notice any changes in your body? If so, what were they?
- How did your thoughts or emotions shift when you visualized this event?
- Were you able to freeze this image in your mind, and get in touch with as many details of this event as possible?
- Were you able to draw an imaginary line between the edge of your comfort zone and this other person?
- When the "line was crossed," was it physical, verbal, mental or emotional in nature?
- How did you feel when you saw this imaginary line separating you from this person or situation?
- What did it feel like to meet your edge in this way?
- Were there changes in your body or feelings? If so, what were they?
- Were you able to move your imaginary line back a few feet, to a more comfortable place?
- If so, how did your feelings shift?
- How did the physical sensations in your body shift?
- And how did the situation play out with your new boundaries in place?

- Do you feel that you can bring this new awareness into your waking life?
- Were you able to capture everything that came up for you in the meditation during the Follow Up Exercise?
- When you did your Off the Mat Practice, were you able to feel yourself in your body at least once per day, even if it was only for a minute?
- Did you notice additional issues that seemed to be connected to your boundaries?
- Did you notice any moments during the week that really pressed you against your edge?
- If so, what were these moments like? What did they have in common?
- Did you notice any raw feelings when you were pressed against your edge this week?
- If not, how were your feelings affected?
- Were you able to notice your boundaries a bit more, or where you've established them so far in your life?
- Do you think your boundaries might have a link with your weight?
- If so, how do you think they might be related?
- Were you able to practice with shifting your boundaries to be a bit more comfortable?
- If so, how did that feel, both physically and emotionally?
- When you shifted your boundaries, even if it was very slightly, did you notice anyone treating you differently? If so, how so?
- Were you able to begin noticing your edge a little sooner each time?
- How did that feel to you?
- Were you able to say "enough" to yourself, and draw a boundary right there in the present moment? Why or why not?
- When you did the Extend Your Practice with Story exercise, were you able to bring to mind a time from your early life in which you didn't feel respected?
- If so, how did it affect your mind?
- How did it affect your body?
- Were you able to see how this instance affected your dreams going forward?
- Were you able to see how this might have divided your body from your mind?

- Were you able to get in touch with a similar event from your adolescent years?
- When you added to your personal narrative, were you able to include lots of details, such as sights, sounds, smells, colors and textures?
- Did any unexpected memories come up when you added to your narrative?
- Were you able to bring to mind a time from your adult life in which you didn't feel respected for who you were?
- How did it feel to get in touch with your limits, and to experiment with removing them from your life?
- Finally, how are you feeling about yourself at this moment?

As you bear these prompts in mind, allow your mind to free you to write all you need to write. If you've had a bad day, or a trying afternoon, or a distracting morning, take this time for yourself. Let yourself push practical concerns aside for the moment so you can move more deeply into your inner core. Let your stories and experience flow out of you like a river. If your Internal Editor trips you up, simply flow around it, over it, or through it. Your stories have the power of water. They can fill the space of your life, wear obstacles down, and even heal old wounds.

When you've come to the end of whatever you need to say right now, sit with your feelings for a few moments. Notice your body, and the sensations it's experiencing. Notice your mind, and its busyness (or stillness) now. Notice how you feel pulled in one direction or another, depending on the circumstances of this present moment.

You Are the Prophet

The poet Jalal al-Din Rumi began his life in what is now Afghanistan, to a father who was a jurist and Sufi preacher. His family moved frequently during his lifetime in the 13th century, due to political unrest in the region. He was married at eighteen and had a son, but continued to seek the answers to life's many spiritual questions.

It wasn't until October of 1244, when he met a whirling dervish named Shamsuddin of Tabriz, also called Shams, that he began to question the spiritual teachings he had carried with him since his youth. Shams did not observe the *Shariah*, or holy law of Islam, which

Rumi had followed all his life, and was soon spending a great deal of time with Rumi, showing him another, more mystical way of looking at the world.

But Shams left Rumi's life almost as soon as he entered it. Rumi searched for his friend for many years, writing poems of intense longing. He began to understand the concept of spiritual love, and applied it fervently to his friend and God alike. And none of it would have been possible if he had not known Shams, and not allowed his worldview to be shattered in his presence.

Rumi's poetry can teach us a lot about how to allow ourselves to become inspired by the people and forces in our lives. Too often, we are taught to be distant, jaded and therefore complacent in our responses to life's wonders. Not often enough do we spool out our emotional rope, take chances, allow ourselves to be as fully vulnerable as we can as humans. The hunger we feel is often translated, without much thought, into a hunger for food. So we stuff our mouths until they're full, and never really feel satisfied.

I love Rumi's story, because it's applicable to so many areas of our lives. All of us are born into a certain family, at a certain time. We grow up with siblings, in a particular place, and all of this combines to form our experience. We go to school. We graduate and enter the workforce. We start and end relationships. We live, as fully as we can.

All of us have run into a person like Shams. From our perspective, he or she may look crazy or demented, incapable of toeing the lines drawn by "ordinary" society. This person may seem scary or fascinating by turns. The common denominator is that there is a connection with the divine in this person, a striving to reach beyond what we see and hear each day, a longing to connect the seeking parts of ourselves to God.

This may not seem to have an immediate connection with losing weight and trying to achieve your best body. But this program is designed to take you through some common emotional disruptions that often occur during any weight loss journey, and then to spark your imagination to go farther, if you so desire. Shams came into Rumi's life to connect him with the deepest parts of himself, and to have a reason to write down his stories, in poems of exquisite beauty. He also began to dance, as a way of reinforcing this connection with the divine. *Dhikr* is an Arabic word that means *remembrance* or *memory*, and was thought to be the rhythmic expression of this divine connection. For Rumi, there was no separation between his mind and his body, his body and God. The same is true for you.

The mistaken belief about losing weight is that it's temporary. We believe we'll go on a diet, lose the desired number of pounds, and then suddenly stop eating that way. Everyone will want us, and think we're attractive and funny and they'll be unable to imagine life without us. Men or women will fall at our feet. We'll become successful and wealthy overnight, too.

It's as if we believe time will stop when the weight has disappeared. We'll exist in a little bubble of timelessness, and nothing will be able to infringe on our new hotness. Our minds stop when we imagine the new clothing we'll buy, or the swimsuit we'll wear next summer. But what happens to our minds and bodies when we've achieved our goals?

If we met a goal and then stopped doing what's worked, we'd probably stop exercising for the calories it burns, completely overlooking the cardiovascular and other health benefits it brings. We'd stop drinking too much, or using drugs for a week or two, until the behavior had changed, and then go right back to using them. It sounds silly, doesn't it? But it's exactly what we do with the food that goes into our bodies. We don't eat to fit into a certain size swimsuit, but to nourish every part of our existence.

Keeping Up Appearances

For many of us, losing weight may be a way of making ourselves attractive to others. Almost every aspect of our culture teaches us that we're no one unless others desire us. We may buy into the myths that we'll end up alone and unloved, or just without the emotional support we all need to live successfully. But why are we so easily manipulated?

Advertising, and the people who create it, study human weaknesses, and learn to exploit them with focused and deliberate intention. All of us are programmed, deep within our DNA, to fear anything that could potentially kill us, and so we internalize those fears, and direct them against anything that seems threatening. This includes the fear of being alone, or not having the love we need, not just to enjoy a quality of life, but to actually survive. Fear of losing what we need to survive (in this case, social groupings) has a way of making us fall right into line, and buy whatever's being sold. It also has a way of reinforcing our interdependence, if we let it.

Rumi's tale reminds us that we can be the safest and sanest folks around, but that will never protect us entirely. For most of his life, Rumi did all the right things. He followed the traditional religious teachings of his father. He got married and had a family. He formed positive connections with his community. But none of that could protect his life from being upended by the decidedly unwelcome presence of Shams in his life.

Just as you're writing your personal narrative each week, spilling out your innermost thoughts and feelings, Rumi was forced to confront all that didn't work about his life when Shams came in. You may have stepped on the scale one day to see a number you didn't like. You may have found that your clothes no longer fit. Or perhaps someone said something hurtful to you. Instead of allowing these instances to stop you in you tracks, or drive you into a self-protective inner space, see them for what they are. The number on the scale is Shams. The clothing that no longer fits is also Shams. And the unkind comment is Shams, blasting into your life to shock you back in touch with yourself.

Just as Rumi did, learn to throw off appearances for the sake of others. Learn to contact that soft, inner part of you. Let it sing out with longing for the person you want to become.

Trusting Your Gut

As we've seen in previous chapters, people who tend to carry weight often find it hard to establish and reinforce strong boundaries. They may have a history with habitual boundary transgressors, or just not have the emotional tools yet to understand why this feels bad. Our bodies are truly miraculous in that they give us all the signals we will ever need in order to survive. If a certain food isn't good for our digestive systems, our intestines rumble with displeasure, or we might experience a stomachache. If we're fearful of someone, with no real reason, we'll feel "butterflies" in our stomachs.

If you plan to adjust your food plan so it brings maximum nutrition while still allowing for healthy weight loss, you may want to start by just cutting calories. This is a time-tested way of losing weight, by burning more calories than you take in. But if you develop trust in yourself, including your body, you may find that you're able to learn what your body wants and needs without undue help from diet "experts."

Your gut has been developed over literally millions of years. As humans, we have adapted to the food sources available to us, as well as the climate and other factors. Our bodies contain that genetic code, in addition to the codes of our families, our ethnicity, and even the regions we live in. Our cells "remember" all of this, and react to what we put into our bodies accordingly. That's why a model may be able to eat certain foods that make you ill, and a movie star may be able to keep trim by working out twenty minutes a day when it takes thirty (or sixty or ninety) for you.

Rather than cursing genetics, which only depends and extends the self-hatred sometimes born from being heavy, I've found that adopting a lifelong program of eating a balanced diet, exercising as part of your weekly routine, and using spiritual development techniques like meditation, is the ticket to my best body. Genetics will always play a part in how I look, and that's as it should be. Self-acceptance, no matter what size you are, is undeniably huge.

I know it doesn't sound glamorous. I'm not promising a fifty-pound weight loss in the next three days, or a vacation on some exotic island. I didn't name my plan after a hot U.S. city, nor have celebrities I've never met write testimonials for my book. But I do want you to accept that you already have all the power you will ever need inside you, to change your body if you so desire, or just bring greater health to your life. By combining the physical, emotional, mental and spiritual aspects of your life, you dare to claim that power for yourself, and refuse to give it up to whatever trend is hot this month.

It all starts with trusting your gut. If your throat burns, there's a reason. If you have a stomachache, or your intestines are rumbling, chances are your body is trying to tell you something. Take the time, no matter how busy you are. Listen.

Grounding Yourself Without Food

Ask anyone who has a weight problem and you're likely to get the same answer. Food is wonderful. Its flavors, textures and, most of all, associations drive us to consume it for our nutrition needs and just for fun sometimes. Over the past ten or so years, the "foodie" movement, along with the creation of the Food Network on television, have made food even more prevalent in our culture and in our minds.

While it's important to eat a balanced diet, it's easy to get "hooked" on the idea of food, and become obsessed with its creation, preparation and of course, consumption. As we've explored in previous chapters, becoming hooked, or caught up in the mental aspects of anything, begins to fray the connection between our minds and bodies. So it's important to develop other ways of grounding yourself without food.

A daily meditation practice is one of my favorite methods for doing this. As we've explored, meditation establishes your connection with the earth through your legs, thighs, ankles and feet, if you're sitting on a cushion or mat, or through the bottoms of your feet, if you're sitting in a chair. During walking meditation, our connection with the earth is re-established every time we take another step.

Exercise is another crucial way of cementing your connection with the earth. I happen to like exercising, but understand people who don't. Ever since gym class, throwing those God-forsaken rubber balls at one another, many of us have adopted a "don't go there" attitude when it comes to exercising. We feel that we have to be talented athletes or we'll be deemed uncoordinated. Also, when trying to lose weight, we may believe that we have to do the highest calorie-burning activities, which can also bring out those fears of coordination and do more harm than good if they're accompanied by injuries or detrimental health conditions. Nonsense. These days, exercise can be as simple as walking, dance, stretching (yoga), or moving meditation (tai chi). No matter what your fitness level, there's a safe and effective way to start exercising.

Other great ways of keeping this connection to the earth alive is to visit it on a regular basis. By this I mean getting out in nature as much as you can. Depending on where you live, you may be able to go hiking on a regular basis (hey, it's great exercise as well), help a local nature organization clear trails or plant trees, tend a personal or community garden, even one on your windowsill. Use your meditation practice of connecting your senses to extend yourself into the natural world.

If you honor your connection with the earth in this way, please bring all of your intention with you. It's so easy, when we're all so busy and stressed out, to bring that into the natural world. And that's fine, if you need nature to help calm you down. But you'll derive greater benefits by simply being in your body as you walk through a secluded grove of ancient trees, scale the stony face of a mountain, or sink your hands into loamy dirt to pat it around delicate flower bulbs. Bring your meditation off the mat as you feel yourself moving through space, as you stand still in wonder, and as you feel the magnetic pull of gravity through your feet.

The earth is always there for us. It may sound corny, but it's true. It can lend us its strength when we're feeling fragile, and provide for us when we're feeling weak. When we undertake a program of losing weight and achieving our best bodies, we will need all the support we can get. Our mates, friends and family members are an integral part of this journey inward. Finding creative ways to connect yourself to the grounding energy of the earth without food is yet another way to find that needed support at a time you may need it most.

Fending Off Disease & Addiction

Learning to ground yourself without food is also important when it comes to understanding how your body uses what it gets from food to help your body function. We all know that if we don't eat, we die. We all know that we need vitamins and minerals typically found in our food to live healthy lives. But we seldom give thought to the fact that the food we eat can also rob our bodies of these benefits, and actually cause harm.

The main function of anyone's body is to keep itself alive. That's it. Simple enough. Your body wants you to live, even when you're telling it, by feeding it junk, that you don't want to live. In this way, many of us are in constant battle with the very things looking out for our survival. No diet commercial is ever going to put it that way.

The more we go on like this, slowly poisoning ourselves by eating whatever's on the table or within arm's reach, the more our bodies lose faith in us. I don't mean to anthropomorphize them, but physiologically, there are systems in the body that begin to override what we're doing, so our survival is ensured. One of these is the accumulation of weight, which acts almost like a softening barrier between us and these bodily systems.

Our spirits become sick when this happens. We begin to want less, to reach out less, and to isolate ourselves in our minds. Even if we have active social lives and people calling us all the time, we still fall victim to this thinking. And to counter it, we may display dishonesty, sadness, grieving, victimization, cheating or lying. We may be the happiest and most honest people around, but when we allow our spirit to become ill in this way, we often don't notice that we're falling into these behaviors because our connection with ourselves has been broken.

We may also become sicker on a physical level. As our bodies are neglected and fall into disrepair, they will compensate by trying to force certain systems into overdrive. If we're not getting enough vitamins from our food or supplementation, for example, our systems will try to leech these vitamins from other places. And if our spirits aren't there to support us, in every possible way, we will tend to become sicker faster, and our illnesses will last far longer than if our spirits were truly engaged with creating a healthy and satisfactory life for us.

Addictions are another way we can succumb to illness in the body and spirit. If we create a situation in which we don't care for our bodies, or don't feel we have the adequate money, food, or support to do so, we're broadcasting an energetic message – *You don't have to care for me, either*. This creates a shaky foundation upon which many of us decide to build.

Everything's fine, right? We go along with our lives, reaching for our goals, only to be surprised again and again that they do not come to fruition, or not in the way we'd hoped. That relationship didn't work out, that job didn't come through, and our weight's still going up.

What's going on?

This is fertile ground for addictions, because whatever we've convinced ourselves to expect isn't happening. It can't happen, because we've created an unworkable situation. But our conscious minds don't know that. Instead, we begin to believe the terrible things our inner critics tell us. We begin to believe we're unlovable, unsuccessful and worthy of nothing. We begin to rely on food, exercise, relationships, drugs, alcohol, sex or gambling in order to feel appreciated. We slip, a little more each day, into the arms of a false lover.

In trying to run before we've learned to walk, we've forged ahead without giving ourselves what we'll need in terms of personal support, meaning the mental and emotional tools we'll need to navigate the world. And in some cases, we weren't ready to do that. We were raised in our households of origin, and may have never had the opportunity to develop these tools. That's why it's so imperative to do it now, or at least in tandem with any weight loss program. Building self-esteem, coping tools and strength of character are crucial, I have found. If you know who you are, what you're willing to do and, more importantly, what you're not willing to do, you've already given yourself the powerful position in any given situation.

Slowing ourselves down, looking inward on a regular basis and searching for the connections between our behaviors and the internal (and sometimes physiological) mechanisms that control them help to break the grip of addictions. After all, addictions depend on all of us to remain unaware. They ask us to let them drive our lives, while we sit in the passenger seat with a blindfold on. They need us to be as complacent and easy as possible, so they can retain control of our lives.

In my work, I've noticed many heavy people carrying one or more cross-addictions. Sexual addicts may eat too much. Gamblers may never eat, in order to spend more on their addiction. Food addicts may be suffering from a dependence on drugs they use to help them stay awake or try to lose weight. Placing more importance on these relationships requires constant gut checking, sometimes literally and sometimes metaphorically. When you choose to keep the power for yourself, addictions have nothing to hold onto. Eventually, with constant attention and awareness, they let go and drop away.

The Relationship of "Stuck" Energy to Weight Loss

I've met a fair number of people who seem to defy all scientific odds. They've adopted better diets, cut their calories and increased their calorie-burning exercise. But still, their weight doesn't budge, or not much. According to conventional wisdom, they should be losing weight at a steady rate of about 1.5-3 pounds per week by doing these things.

The more we understand about the body, the more doctors and scientists can approach the question of losing weight. But why are we seeing more and more of this? Why are humans retaining weight around their midsections more than any other part of the body? Some of this must be genetic. But all of it? Not likely.

Many naturopaths conclude that diseases of the spirit, including "stuck" energies, are contributing to this phenomenon. Humans are, essentially, batteries. Each of us is charged with energy that runs through us in meridians, or lines that run from the very top of our heads to the bottom of our feet. This energy is required for all normal bodily functions like eating and sleeping, urinating, sweating and defecating. It controls our metabolism and our emotions, and assists in the breakdown and elimination of all we eat.

But if we don't move our energy on a regular basis, by exercising, stretching, thinking, meditating and constantly challenging ourselves, we run the risk of letting our energies get "stuck" in various parts of our bodies. This is not literal; you cannot see stuck energy on an x-ray. But if you cultivate self-awareness, you may be able to feel it. You may seem out of sorts, or irritable for no reason. You may have an unexplained pain or heavy sadness. Or you may feel angry and furious with the world, not understanding why. These are all signs that you may have stuck energy that needs to be moved along if you're going to lose weight.

Hinduism and other belief systems believe that all of our energies are controlled by the chakras, which are imaginary wheels placed on the body in seven locations:

- The 1st chakra is located near the anus and perineum. Its color is red, and it rules survival and self-preservation.
- The 2nd chakra is located near the abdomen, lower back and genitals. Its color is orange, and it rules reproduction and sexuality.
- The 3rd chakra is located near the stomach and digestive system. Its color is yellow, and it rules ego and self-definition.
- The 4th chakra is located near the heart. Its color is green, and it rules love, self-acceptance and our social identity.
- The 5th chakra is located near the throat. Its color is bright blue, and it rules communication, creativity and self-expression.
- The 6th chakra is located near the third eye, in the middle of the forehead. Its color is dark blue, and it rules second sight and our ability to self reflect.
- The 7th chakra is located near the top of the head. Its color is purple, and it rules our connection with God and higher beings, as well as self-knowledge.

Much has been written about the chakras and their relationship to our mental, emotional and spiritual wellbeing, and I believe we're only beginning to scratch the surface of how these energies affect our day-to-day health. My work with people healing from early traumas, or writing the stories pertinent to their lives in an effort to heal, has made it clear to me that somehow, we must all keep these subtle energies moving smoothly, without interruption.

The most helpful modalities for removing stuck energy seem to be those that derive organically from the source. For example, if you're a gym-phobic person, it won't make much sense to suggest you start pumping iron. If you hate traveling, it won't do much good for you to pretend you do. But if you're able to adopt a modality that takes into account your likes and dislikes, fears and joys, you're likely to internalize it on a physical level. Also, you're much more likely to stay with it, which will bring more benefits over time.

Again, a consistent meditation practice is one way to rid your body of stuck energies, as well as yoga or tai chi. All of these disciplines work with the subtle energies of the body and make sure they stay balanced and healthy, which provides a foundation for weight loss, a new exercise program, or even adopting a new way of dealing with emotional issues.

But if you're not drawn to these activities, you can still make sure energy doesn't become an obstacle to your weight loss journey. A former client I will call Rebecca recently lost her sister to breast cancer. They were very close, and Rebecca contacted me to help remember her sister by co-authoring a book about their lives together. They'd grown up in rural Maine, in a kind of Louisa May Alcott crossed with Steven King childhood, filled with ghosts and lighthouses and storytelling. I was looking forward to the project, because it seemed like very rich and fertile ground for a memoir.

But before we even got started, Rebecca started calling me on a regular basis to express her fears. Did her sister want her to expose and possibly profit from their shared childhood? Was she doing her wrong by making light of their time together? After all, her sister had lived through several troubled years of unhappiness. Often, she was without direction and/or suicidal.

At the same time, Rebecca was trying to lose weight using a popular diet plan. She had quit smoking when her sister died because doctors told her their shared genetics, combined with her smoking and unhealthy eating habits, could put her at risk for getting breast cancer as well. She was irritable and began having strange and colorful dreams she deemed prescient. But Rebecca had a sedentary job at a bank, in which she processed loan applications all day. The job was fine, she said, a bit boring, but fine for covering her expenses.

She was about ready to give up on the project completely when I suggested we take a walk one day to talk about whether or not she really wanted to continue. We walked up a steep hill in the Santa Monica Mountains, just taking our time. After a few moments, I could tell she was thinking about her sister, about their lives together. Her gaze was cast downward, watching her footsteps on the path. We were silent for a few minutes.

When we reached the summit, we stood at the ridge-line, looking out over the ocean. It was preternaturally beautiful, with the sun sparkling over the rich azure water.

"I forgot how good walking feels," she confessed. "Maybe that's silly to say."

"Not at all."

We stood there, just taking in the view for a few minutes, then sat on the ground talking. She told me about her fears for the book project, but mentioned that she was feeling a lot better about it now. "Maybe it's the nice day, the weather …" she trailed off.

I have always felt that what changed Rebecca's mind that day was the walk itself. She was out of breath on the way up the hill, but had a dogged look on her face, the same look that had gotten her through those tough days in the hospital, holding her sister's hand. When she emerged at the summit, I could tell she was proud of herself for having achieved it. But there was something more underneath, as if she were making a new promise to herself.

We went forward with the book project and Rebecca chose to keep walking, making loops around the blocks in her neighborhood and then walking around a track at a local high school. She began to lose weight quite easily, and her mood began to change. Her memory improved as well, and stories about her sister began to tumble out. Maybe it's oversimplifying to attribute all of this to a walk up a mountain, but that is the moment when everything changed for Rebecca. That's when she realized she could tell this story without upsetting the ghost of her sister, and that her own life could change as well, with some adjustments to her energies.

In time, she remembered that she and her sister had loved dancing, and that they had often danced together, just to be silly, when they were children. She decided to take a "real" dance class, as she called it, and enjoys dancing to this day, whether it's silly or serious.

There are as many modalities for ridding the body of stuck energy as there are stars in the sky. Whatever your mind is drawn to at this transitional time of your life, explore. Whatever your head tells you you can't do, or you shouldn't do, check out. It's not enough anymore, in our fast-paced, sophisticated world, to say you can't, or you won't, or you haven't. It's time to say you will, and you can, and you have, even if it's scary.

Rewriting the Story of Your Life

The purpose for writing this book has always been to empower people with the gift of healing, using something everyone already has – his or her own stories. So my final advice to anyone reading this book is to take the personal narrative you have been writing over eight weeks, as well as the lessons you've learned through moving all of the Follow Up and Off the Mat Exercises, and to begin the process of rewriting your life.

Writing is magical, not just in the fairy-dust, Harry Potter sense, but in the "ability to change reality" sense. For thousands of years, priests, priestesses and other holy figures have used writing to bring good fortune to their tribes and cultures, and to keep evil away. In the same way, each of us can use the power of our own personal stories to extend our healing as far into the future as we can imagine. People who follow the Wiccan religion often use writing to cast spells. And millions of people all over the world talk to diaries and journals each day, asking for help in sorting out the events of their lives.

When we write down our intentions, they begin to become solidified. Energetically, we're linking our intentions to the intentions of the rest of the Universe. In a sense, we're catching onto a huge wave, by merging our energies with those of the larger body. Sometimes, being part of something this large is frightening to people. Each of us likes to feel in control of our lives and our destinies. Others feel comforted that being part of this stream protects them.

In a way, we can hedge our bets against an inconsistent world by rewriting our stories every day. We become more aware of what we have been through by remembering our past and committing it to paper (or recorder). We honor what we have been through by memorializing it. And we have a chance to "do it over again" by rewriting how we would have preferred to have it happen in our lives. Of course, this doesn't mean that that schoolyard bully didn't beat you up at recess, but it does mean you can begin the process of digging out and releasing any old, negative self-beliefs buried as a result of this incident.

Rewriting the stories of our lives connects us to the events as they happened in real time. But since the act of writing engages the right, or creative side of the brain, we "fool" our systems into healing and acceptance by using this tool. Rewriting begins with knowing, very deeply and intimately, who you are. It's not as simple as understanding what your favorite color is, who your friends are, or what your favorite meal consists of. It's a far more arduous process, of digging out, remembering and holding up to the light all those boring, embarrassing, painful and distinctly human memories we all have. It also demands that you be willing to be authentic with everything you find, and I mean *everything*. If you find yourself wishing your parents were dead, that is real. It doesn't mean you should kill them, or that you will. But it means there is something there to be looked at, examined, and hopefully released.

Looking at these memories is sometimes unpleasant. Stay with it. Holding them up to the light makes us want to flinch. But we must keep looking. Applying our hard-won wisdom and authentic attention to them may be harder than anything we've ever done. But in order to bring true healing, the kind that sticks around far longer than it takes the next popular self-help book to come out, we must apply this wisdom, every day, even if we only have five conscious minutes.

Our stories make us human. They provide our moral framework, and connect us to each other in ways we may be completely unaware of on a moment-to-moment basis. But working with your stories, and learning how to rewrite them to facilitate healing, or help you reach seemingly unreachable goals, will become a powerful tool in your arsenal. You never have to look outside yourself anymore, though you may choose to work with others in storytelling workshops or groups. You never have to rely on others to do what you want them to do, because everything you need is right inside you.

Go ahead. Tell your stories. We're all out here, waiting and listening.

Meditation

For our final meditation, we'll spend some time examining how we can ground ourselves in ways that don't involve over-eating, or subverting our goals for achieving our best bodies. We'll see how each of us has the choice, in any given moment, to choose methods that will keep us on track, or send us hurtling off our chosen path, and begin to understand how these choices have far more serious ramifications than our immediate satisfaction.

Coming back Down to Earth may require deep personal awareness, as well as the ability to bring crystal-clear wisdom to any given situation. After all, we cannot always control our eating, or even what's available for us to eat. Sometimes, our jobs or other responsibilities leave us with no time to work out or engage in any real stress relief. Only by knowing ourselves extremely well can we begin to remove anything that stands in our way of achieving our stated goals.

This week's meditation begins the process of taking that wisdom and sending it out into the world. You have worked very hard to attain it and develop it. Now it's time to share it with others, directly or indirectly.

• Begin by going to your meditation space, and closing the door if possible. This will give you the privacy you need to close out any distractions and really focus on your needs and goals. Make sure you've brought along your notebook and writing implement, or mini-cassette recorder, if you've chosen to record your experience in this way.

• Then bring your body into your preferred meditation posture. Sit on the floor, on a mat or cushion, with your legs crossed underneath your body for support. As you inhale deeply, let your shoulders follow your breath. They will naturally move upward and slightly back, without you having to arch your back or force them into this position.

- As you exhale, let your shoulders stay in this position as your chest falls. Without forcing yourself to become too rigid, retain this upright and dignified meditation posture. As you move through the 7 Points of Posture in your mind, adjust your body so it supports you fully and effortlessly. As a reminder, the 7 Points of Posture are: the seat and legs, the eyes and gaze, the spine, the shoulders, the neck and throat, the mouth and tongue, and the hands.

- Then bring your attention to each of your five senses in turn, connecting each to your meditation. As you focus on your eyes, say "seeing" to yourself. As you focus on your ears, say "hearing" to yourself. As you focus on your mouth, say "tasting" to yourself. As you focus on your nose, say "smelling" to yourself. And finally, as you focus on your hands and fingers, say "touching" to yourself.

- Begin your Base Practice by bringing your attention to your breath as it moves in and out of your body. As you notice thoughts and storylines entering your consciousness, say "thinking" to yourself and let them ride your breath as you breathe out. There's no need to bring any additional feelings to this process, or do anything about the fact that you're having thoughts. Just get used to doing nothing about them but calling them what they are.

- When you become comfortable with the rhythm you've established, take a moment to notice what the tenor of your thoughts is right now. Are you agitated and angry? Sad and lonely? Enthusiastic and happy? Just notice where your mind wants to take you now.

- Bring your attention to your body, moving through each part of yourself from the top to the bottom. See if you're holding tension anywhere. See if any one part seems disjointed, or out of whack with the other parts. If so, hold your attention here for a few breaths, just noticing the quality of this sensation in your body. How does it feel to be in your body right now?

- Now bring to mind an image of your own body. This can be a mirror image, if you can remember what you look like from top to bottom, or even a quick sketch on your mind – whatever works for you. Just hold that image in your mind for your next few breaths, watching the thoughts that come into your mind as you do so.

• What seems to be coming off this body? Can you sense what it needs? This may be very obvious, depending on the image you see in your mind. If it's not so obvious, ask your body what it needs. To yourself, adopt an open and listening posture as you ask your inner self for guidance. Listen as the information is relayed back to you. No matter what you hear, just abide. Keep listening, without judgment.

• When you have a sense of what your body wants and needs, breathe in deeply. As you do, take on all that's hurting your body – any fears, judgments, negative self-beliefs, personal issues, etc. Think of this as dark, black, smoky or hot in nature. Feel it as it enters your throat and lungs and is immediately transmuted into energy. This has no power to harm you in real life. It's a symbolic exercise to help you dialogue with your own body, often called *tonglen* meditation.

• As you breathe out again, imagine yourself sending whatever your body needs, straight from your heart. See a beam of light or just a symbolic transfer from you to it. See yourself sending more money, more time at the gym, better food and nutrition, or even someone to compliment your progress, and help you stay on track.

• Keep breathing in and out, taking on the pain, anger or fear of your body with your in breath, and sending light, love, coolness and relief with your out breath. Notice what your mind substitutes each time you do this. Does it stay with the same images each time, or does it shift slightly with each inhalation and exhalation? Keep breathing as you watch your mind try to help you repair any of these old, negative issues still lying within.

• As you continue breathing, check in with your body again. Scan though all the parts of your body from the top to the bottom. What has changed, and what has stayed the same? Are the parts that might have held tension feeling any different now? Has the tension shifted to anywhere new? Have you experienced any new sensations you might not have expected? If so, where are they concentrated?

• Go back to your Base Practice, just watching your breath as it moves in and out of your body and labeling your thoughts as they arise in your mind.

• Now picture a red flower or wheel at the bottom of your body, near your seat. You may see this at the front or back of your body – it doesn't matter. Spin this flower or wheel, seeing it open as it spins.

• Move up a little further, to your lower abdomen. Spin an orange flower or wheel here, watching it open wide as it spins around.

• Then move up to your stomach region. Spin a bright yellow flower or wheel here, watching it open as if warmed by the sun.

• Moving up a little further, to your chest, spin a green flower or wheel. Watch it open as it spins and spins and spins.

• Move up to your throat region now, and spin a bright blue flower or wheel. See the petals open up as it keeps revolving around a central spoke.

• Move up to your third eye region, right between your eyes and a little higher. See a dark blue flower or wheel spinning here, smoothly and endlessly.

• Finally, picture a purple flower or wheel spinning at the very top of your head. See it opening to accept all the Universe has to offer.

• Take a mental step back and see all seven chakras spinning in tandem, from your 1st (red) chakra through your 7th (purple) chakra. Beyond that, see a bright pink field of energy all around you, and then a white light that pulses in protection. These are your etheric bodies, which help keep your lines of communication with the Universe open.

- Breathe in and out five times here, just watching all the aspects of your being coming together. See everything about you vibrating with pure, life energy. Feel yourself in your body. Understand that these energetic forces are at work, all the time, within you.

- Then see your body in your mind's eye, sitting on the floor, mat, cushion or chair. Imagine six strings superimposed over your body, vertically, like the strings of a guitar. Mentally pluck each of the strings in turn, "hearing" each of the sustained notes these bodily strings produce. If you feel one or more of your strings doesn't sound right with the others, adjust it by tightening or loosening as needed.

- When you've tuned your "strings" as much as you'd like, mentally strum all the strings together. Hear the sound your body makes when it's "tuned" properly. Notice the sound as it reaches out into the world, and how it ultimately decays as it travels further and further away from you. This represents your energy and intentions as they move into the world, and establish the path upon which your wishes will return to you.

- As you strum your strings again, see the waves of sound energy moving away from your body. Bring your awareness to all you want to achieve with your body, how you want to look and feel, and how you want to form a new relationship with your body. Feel your energy as it moves out into the world, interacts with the energy of others, and comes back to you, in a perfect circle.

- Check in with your mind now. Are you having any strong thoughts or storylines? If so, what do they look like, or sound like?

- Check in with your body. Move through all your component parts, to see if anything has shifted during your meditation. Are the same tensions or pains there, or have they moved on? Have any new sensations arisen to take their place?

- Let the images in your mind go, and return to your Base Practice. Take five full breaths in and out here, just letting everything go.

When you notice thoughts or storylines in your mind, tap them lightly on the shoulder and say "thinking" to yourself. Let them leave you as you breathe out.

• Come out of the meditation, allowing your normal, waking consciousness to return. Give yourself plenty of extra time as you get up from your meditation and move on to the next task at hand.

Follow Up Exercise

The tendency, when coming out of a meditation session, may be to rush to your notebook and immediately record everything you've just been through. But make sure you've given yourself an adequate break. Get some water if you need to, then sit down with your notebook or mini-cassette recorder. Make sure to find a fresh page and date the entry at the top.

Then take a deep breath. Let your mind bring forward the images and sensations you've recently experienced, rather than resorting to aggressive methods to force it to relinquish what it knows. Don't forget that sometimes, the words you may want to use may not make sense. Your feelings may not "go" with what your thoughts are telling you. Record them anyway. Our bodies are intelligent beings. They are in constant communication with us, and it's our duty to try and set aside the language differences in order to affect a common goal.

As you begin to record your experiences, remember to place special importance on how your emotions were filtered through your body as you moved through each aspect of the meditation. Normally, we're taught to describe our experiences in very "heady" ways, using words that describe our thoughts about what happened, without actually letting the experience permeate us on a physical level. So when you write about how you experienced each aspect of the meditation, including any feelings, memories or snatches of dreams it may have jarred loose, make sure to pay special attention to how your body was affected at each stage.

As always, I'll give you a few writing prompts to get you started:

• As you worked to establish your meditation posture, how did you feel?
• Were any emotions strong in you as you began?

- How did you feel about this being the last week in our program together?
- Has your meditation posture evolved over time, or have you found one that seems to work for you?
- Are you able to stick with the meditation sessions for about 15-20 minutes, shifting your posture as necessary to stay upright and dignified?
- Are you able to recall and work with the 7 Points of Posture pretty easily?
- How has the relationship between your mind and your body evolved since you began this process? How has it stayed the same?
- Are there still areas you'd like to work on as you progress with your meditations?
- How have your senses been affected as you move about in your daily life? How have you incorporated them into the communications you receive from your body?
- If any memories were dislodged as a result of this meditation, what were they?
- Are these memories happy or sad in nature? And how have they affected your mood right now, at this point in time?
- How have your emotions changed from before you started the meditation?
- How have the sensations in your body changed since you started the meditation?
- Was it easy to bring to mind an image of your body, and ask it what it needed?
- Did you receive an answer, or sense, from your body, about what it needs now?
- If so, what does your body need more than anything else?
- As you breathed in all that your body found overwhelming or scary, what did you find? Were the fears and anxieties solid in nature, or all mixed together?
- How did your body seem to react when you did this?
- When you breathed out, sending your body all you thought it needed, how did you feel? What did you send your body?
- When you checked back in with your body, had anything shifted?
- If so, what happened with your body?

- When you started to spin each of your chakras, from the bottom of your body to the top, how did you feel? Was this a new experience for you?
- If so, were you able to see how your energy connects each part of your body to the next?
- Were you able to see how your energy connects your mind with your body as well?
- How did it feel to see yourself as an energetic being?
- How did it feel to see yourself as an upright guitar, with strings?
- Were you able to "tune yourself," and get the sound coming off those strings to sound harmonious to your ears?
- How was your body affected when you did this?
- How was your mind affected?
- What was your first thought when you came out of the meditation?

By now, you're probably used to the routine. Make sure to get down all of your experiences in the meditation as quickly as you can. This is not a race, or to see if you can break some sort of land speed record. Instead, it's meant to help you bypass your Internal Editor, so you're free to record what you've been through in as pure and authentic a way possible.

If this part of the process begins to feel like a chore, remind yourself that you are getting to know yourself. Every time you have wanted someone else to reach out to get to know you better has been an example of this same desire, just in another form. Give yourself some of what you're hoping for, and others are likely to see that you're worth giving to as well. Usually, few people will go out of their way to know you better unless you've take your very valuable time to get to know yourself.

Do your meditation exercises every day of the next week or more you decide to practice with Down to Earth. Giving yourself just 10-20 minutes, and more if you can find the time, proves to your spouse, your boss, your family and the Universe that you are truly worth knowing in a more intimate way. Don't forget to bring your notebook and mini-cassette recorder with you, so you can make sure the experiences you capture are the freshest and most honest you have to offer at this time. If you give yourself the time, there's nothing you can't achieve!

Off the Mat Practice

Many people who carry extra weight tend to ground themselves with food, as we have seen in this chapter. But if you want to become the prophet in your own life, truly empowered as Rumi was, it's important to find other ways to do this. Continuing to practice with ways to bring us back down to earth, or to re-connect our minds to our bodies, may reveal ways in which we've created mental obstacles to our own success, or internalized issues or "weights" which are not ours to carry.

This week, try to notice instances when you feel flighty or ungrounded. This may occur in your body, such as when your stomach feels filled with butterflies, or when you find it hard to concentrate, or focus on the work you're doing. It may occur when you're driving, and can't seem to remember where you're going, or when you've lost some important papers at home. And it may even happen when your mind is so crowded with the things you need to do that you forget something simple, like a co-worker's name.

However it manifests in your life, just notice it. Try not to harden your mind about it, or force yourself to endure a torturous mental exercise in order to remember more. This is your mind's (or your body's) way of telling you that you've reached your limit. Discovering these moments can help you see where you allow yourself to become uncomfortably ungrounded.

Then notice how you feel in these moments. How do they effect your emotions and your body? Are you tempted to eat more at these times, or to eat more than you would ordinarily? Do you have certain cravings in these moments and, if so, what kinds of food do you crave? Note anything significant in your notebook or mini-cassette recorder.

As you begin to bring your attention to these moments of feeling groundless, also begin to notice moments when you're overly concerned with your appearance. For instance, do you go overboard in buying clothing, so you're always perfectly turned out? Do you decide to do or say things by considering what others will think or feel above all? Or is your sole reason for wanting to lose weight how others will treat you, when all is said and done?

Each time you notice one of these moments, just sit with it. Feel the emotions that move through your body as energy. Feel yourself in your body and let yourself just rest there, knowing that every time you allow yourself to become closer to your inner being, the more you can remove the obstacles standing in the way of your success.

As you notice these moments, think about how you would prefer them to be. For instance, you may not want to orient your world just around yourself, but is there a way to share important parts of your life with others without losing yourself in the process? How can you develop tools to help you identify which moments are best for speaking up, and which ones are better for listening? And how can you begin to make decisions that make your quality of life better without negatively affecting those around you?

Don't forget to feel yourself in your body at least once per day while you are still and resting, and while you're in motion, either walking, running, stretching or something else entirely. As a quick exercise, feel the pull of gravity on your body, not in a negative way but as a warm, solid grounding force that helps to keep you balanced and sane. Feel your feet as they anchor you to the ground. Feel the embrace of the Earth's atmosphere as it keeps you upright and mobile.

If you want to take your Off the Mat Practice a bit further, try to notice how you mentally override what your body may be telling you. This is very tricky to spot sometimes, so do your best until it comes a bit more naturally. It may be found in moments when your body is craving a particular kind of food. You may find that a craving for spinach is really your body telling you that you need more iron, or a craving for meat a call for more protein. Do you allow your body what it needs in these moments, or do you "shout it down" by mentally telling it to sit down and shut up, or feeding it whatever is cheapest, can be had around the house, or has the fewest calories?

On the other hand, do you find yourself eating food that's supposed to be good for you, even if you suffer gas, digestive pain, intestinal cramps or diarrhea? In that case, even if a food is allegedly good for us as a species, it may not be good for you. Further investigation may be needed to determine the best foods to nurture your unique body.

Work on trusting your gut a little more each day. This may be physical, as discussed above, or emotional, such as when your body may be trying to give you signals about a person you meet, or about a situation you find yourself in, at work or in your personal life. Your body, no matter what shape it's currently in, is a perfectly tuned machine, capable of telling you all you need to know about what it needs. If you need to become more attuned to how it's communicating with you, spend some more time listening. After all, it's one of the most powerful tools we possess for acquiring new information, and helping to implement it in our lives.

Extend Your Practice with Story

You began this program nine weeks go, as a support system to achieving your best body. Your personal narrative, added to every week, has shown you that your thoughts, feelings and bodily sensations aren't just intricately linked. They're crucial to removing obstacles to your success, and to moving forward along your chosen path to fruition. Last week, we explored how the concept of Enough had been involved in your struggles with losing weight so far. No doubt you've had your own thoughts, feelings and memories that came up as a result of these exercises.

This week, we'll start by reading over what you've written so far. Please take as long as you need. Some people may have several dozen pages now, while others will have just a few. It depends on how worthy you feel about what your mind and body tell you, and how important you think they are to express. Remember to respect the person you were when you wrote these words, whether they came from week 1 or week 7. Resist the impulse to "correct" anything, even if you find a spelling mistake. There's plenty of time for that later, should you decide you want to use these writings to craft a short story or memoir later on.

Then find a fresh page in your notebook, or an unrecorded section of tape on your mini-cassette recorder. If you need to change the batteries in your recorder, go ahead and do that now. Spend a few minutes just centering yourself, and letting all the mundane details of your day float away from you. Take a few deep breaths. Begin to tune in to your inner life, vibrant and existing on its own currents.

Then begin to think about your life now. Are you the prophet of your own life, or have you allowed someone or something else to assume that role? Begin to write as you think about how you envisioned your life to be when you were younger. How have you achieved the goals you set out for yourself and how have you veered off course? What part of these early goals had to do with losing weight and achieving your best body?

Continue to the next paragraph as you think about how you Keep Up Appearances. Are you so afraid of what others have to say that you don't even eat around them, and instead save all your eating for when you're in private? Are you obsessed about the slightest gain or loss in weight? Do you weigh yourself more than once per day, in an effort to feel better about yourself? Let your pen take down whatever's in your mind, surpassing the grip of the Internal Editor and just letting it rip.

Then think about how your body "talks" to you. Everyone's different, so just sit with your body now and see if it's trying to tell you anything. Have you ever eaten a particular food and had an immediate bodily reaction? Hives? An upset stomach? Nausea? Write about this instance. What did you do after this happened? Were your emotions affected in any way? If it was a favorite food of yours, did you eat it again, or stay away from it? How do you listen to your gut and how do you override it? What circumstances tend to accompany these times?

Would you say you're a person that trusts your gut? How has this made itself noticeable for you, perhaps even today as you went about the business of your life? How does your body react when it wants you to stop eating? When it wants you to eat? When it wants you to feed it a particular kind of food? How does it tell you it's tired or sad? How does it tell you it's happy?

Keep writing. If you're a person struggling to find out what your best body might look and feel like, how have you imagined it in your mind? Have you struggled with trying to ground yourself when life becomes stressed? If so, how have you done that? In what type of instances have you been successful and in what instances have you not been successful? Take some time to really think about this one, then write down whatever your mind sees.

Have you been able to find ways to ground yourself without food? Which ways work for you? Which ones seem silly or contrived? And which ones simply don't even begin to help? Pick one way and keep writing about it for a bit. How does performing this activity make you feel on a physical level? Elated and silly? Dull and tired? Sluggish? Dreamy? Or something else?

Go a bit deeper. Think about how you feel on a physical level when you do this activity. Does it make you feel stronger? More muscular? Lighter on your feet, or more graceful? Or something else? Really try to get inside your body here, then tie the physical experience to the emotions you feel when you're doing it.

Keep that pen going, or your voice speaking into your mini-cassette recorder. This is the most important thing for you to be thinking about now, and the most important thing you could be doing for yourself. Include even the smallest details your mind's eye brings up. It doesn't mater if it doesn't make sense with what you're writing now. Any small bit of information becomes useful in time – let me tell you from experience.

Do you sometimes feel as if your energy is stuck? If so, how has that manifested in your life? Does your physical energy flag? Are you disinterested in the events of your life? Have you adjusted around this phenomenon, thinking that it will never change, or have you taken steps to change it? If so, what steps have you taken and why? Give some thought to the steps you've taken which have proven successful for you. What do they seem to have in common, and how are they different from one another? Do you notice a pattern of activities you're drawn towards?

Each word you write, each sentence, brings you closer to the person you are now. It's easy to say we know who we are, but each of us is so complex, it's easy to lose sight of *all* we are. So give some thought to your life going forward. Where do you want to go from here? How do you want to use the tools you learned by reading this book? How can they help you to adopt a real lifestyle change that can bring years of healing into your life, instead of a 3-6 month diet, which brings starvation, then over-eating, then disappointment?

Rewrite the story of your life here, just the first part. How would you have preferred your life go before this point in time? Obviously, you won't have time to write all of it down in this moment, but hit the high points, or the ones that have bothered you for the longest time. When you were younger, your life wasn't under your control most of the time. Which decisions made by other people colored your life in a positive way? Which decisions caused the most damage to you, and require the most healing?

Start a new paragraph and write about how you would prefer your life to be in the present. Remember, writing is magic. Be very careful with your intentions here. It's not our business to be mean to others or write them out of the picture. But if someone has hurt you, write about how it makes you feel. If someone has taken credit for something you did, write about it from your perspective. And if you feel that something has been taken from you, give it back to yourself on paper. Heal any parts of you that have been left out in the cold, ignored, or pushed aside so you could focus on "more important things."

If you want to be more in touch with your friends, write that down. If you want to attract a new love relationship, put it down. And if you want to be on friendlier terms with food and your body, by all means write that down. But don't forget to put it in the form of a story. Don't just write "I want a new boyfriend." Instead, paint a picture. Describe yourself. What are you wearing? How does your body look? How does it feel to be in your body? How has achieving your best body helped with your self-confidence?

Then move on to the situation. Where are you when you meet this fabulous new person? What are you doing, and how are you feeling? Describe the action of the scene. Then describe this exciting new person. What does he or she look like? What is this person wearing? Is he or she taking part in the same activity as you, or are they doing something different? Is your meeting serendipitous, or planned? Include as many details about what you say, what he or she says, and how you agree to meet again in the future.

Make sure to include information about your feelings as you move through these scenes of your new life, and make sure you relate everything to how your body feels as well. Try not to focus unduly on how others see or treat you. They are free to appreciate you, of course, but try to keep your work confined to how you see yourself, feel about yourself, and want to move forward in your life. Finally, add a paragraph or two on how you believe your new relationship with your body will carry you forward in the world, not just in terms of how you look or who may be attracted to you. Try to think about how this might effect a lifelong change in attitude, both in how you relate to your body and how you care for yourself in the future.

When you feel you've written all there is to say right now, look back at what you've done. You'll probably have about 8-12 paragraphs, and maybe more, depending on how inspired you were. If you think of something else, stop and write it down. Then put down your pen or turn off your mini-cassette recorder.

Take a breath. Get a drink of water if you need to. Then center yourself again and read over what you've written, going all the way back to what you did in week 1. Let your own words sink into your soul. These are your stories, and they have value. Let yourself live through your memories again, laugh or cry when the story demands, and respect the person who was brave enough to share these words with the world.

If you want to, return to your personal narrative each day, or whenever you can find time during the week. Devote yourself to your personal narrative as a practice. Make storytelling a part of your lifestyle going forward.

Speak with your Authentic Voice, and keep speaking. The hunger you feel now is the calling of your soul for deep, spiritual nurturing. That is its food. You will know it when you've come to this point in your practice because you'll feel a profound sense of opening, to yourself, your immediate surroundings, and to all the aspects of your world. Every day you confront the realities of your life, your curiosity will grow. You'll begin to write all your stories, and you simply won't be able to stop.

Resources & Additional Reading

Austin, Dr. James. *Zen and the Brain: Toward an Understanding of Meditation and Consciousness*. Boston, MA: The MIT Press, 1999.

Castillo, Brooke. *If I'm So Smart, Why Can't I Lose Weight?* Charleston, SC: BookSurge Publishing, 2006.

Chodron, Pema. *No Time to Lose: A Timely Guide to the Way of the Bodhisattva*. Boston, MA: Shambhala, 2007.

Dalai Lama. *The Universe in a Single Atom: The Convergence of Science and Spirituality*. New York, NY: Broadway, 2006.

Ginsberg, Allen. Collected Poems 1947-1997. New York, NY: Harper Perennial Modern Classics, 2007.

Ginsberg, Allen. *Howl, and Other Poems*. San Francisco, CA: City Lights Books, 1996.

Kerouac, Jack. *On the Road, 50th Anniversary Edition*. New York, NY: Viking, 2007.

Kerouac, Jack. *The Dharma Bums*. New York, NY: Penguin Classics, 2006.

Mountrose, Phillip & Jane. *The Heart & Soul of EFT and Beyond: A Soulful Exploration of the Emotional Freedom Techniques and Holistic Healing*. San Luis Obispo, CA: Holistic Communications, 2006.

Nhat Hanh, Thich. *The Miracle of Mindfulness*. Danvers, MA: Beacon Press, 1999.

Orbach, Susie. *Fat is a Feminist Issue*. New York, NY: Arrow, 2006.

Orback, Susie. *Susie Orbach on Eating*. New York, NY: Penguin, 2002.

Pert, Candace. *Molecules Of Emotion: The Science Behind Mind-Body*

Medicine. New York, NY: Simon & Schuster, 1999.

Roth, Geneen. *When Food is Love: Exploring the Relationship Between Eating and Intimacy.* New York: Plume, 1992.

Rumi, Jelaluddin. *The Essential Rumi.* New York, NY: Penguin Classics, 2004.

Taylor, Janice. *Our Lady of Weight Loss.* New York, NY: Studio, 2006.

Temes, Roberta. *The Tapping Cure: A Revolutionary System for Rapid Relief from Phobias, Anxiety, Post-Traumatic Stress Disorder and More.* New York: Marlowe & Company, 2006.

Trungpa Rinpoche, Chogyam. *Cutting Through Spiritual Materialism.* Boston, MA: Shambhala, 2002.

Additional Writing Prompts

Make a Vow to Yourself

Spend 10-15 minutes writing about how undertaking this program has renewed your vows towards yourself. How has it made your life seem more important? How has it surprised you? How can making a new vow to yourself every day protect you from sinking into your old habits? Is the process of making vows similar to or different from setting goals in your life?

How You're Defended

Think about how your weight might relate to how you defend yourself against others, or against situations or even institutions. Then write about how your weight has given you permission to *not* take part in your own life, along with ways in which you will take steps to re-engage with whatever you find important. How can you defend yourself without resorting to adding weight?

How Survival Plays a Part

Spend some time thinking about how you may be equating your weight with your need to survive. Have you ever feared going hungry, or starving to death? How has that played out in your "real" life? Has your life been characterized by hardship? How has this affected you as you think about food, eating and your body? Is food a friend or an enemy? What steps can you take to change your relationship with food?

Write About Each Chakra in Turn

Review the information about the chakras in chapter 9, or do some additional research in the library or on the Internet. Then think about how each chakra helps or hinders your progress as it relates to the functioning of your body. Is your attention drawn to any one chakra in particular now? If so, why? Then, starting at your root chakra, take 5-10 minutes to write about each chakra, moving up. How does this chakra's energy make itself known in your life right now? Does concentrating on each chakra in meditation help? Or could you need the help of a professional?

INDEX

INDEX

64, 68, 76, 79, 82-83, 86, 97,
100, 102-103, 108-109, 115,
118, 122, 127, 134, 137, 140-
142, 147, 151, 156, 159-160,
163-165, 171, 173, 180, 182-
184, 189, 194-196, 201

Acknowledgments

The author wishes to thank:

My teachers: His Holiness the Dalai Lama, Chogyam Trungpa Rinpoche, Thich Nhat Hanh and Pema Chodron

My inspiration: Rumi, Allen Ginsberg and Jack Kerouac

My ongoing hope: Candace Pert and all the scientists at the Mind and Life Institute

My reasons: Noel and Bella

About the Author

Alyson Mead's fiction, essays and articles have appeared in over thirty publications, including *Salon.com*, *In These Times*, *Bitch*, *BUST*, *Whole Life Times*, *Punk Planet*, *MS/NBC*, *The Sun*, *AOL*, *IRT*, *The 213*, *Tapestry*, *The Stylus*, and the *New York Daily News*, among others.

She is the author of *Wake up to Your Stories: Using the Art of Personal Narrative to Heal Your Past, Nurture Your Relationships & Ask for What You're Worth*, and has received the Columbine Award for Screenwriting, the Roy W. Dean Filmmaking Grant and a *Writer's Digest* Award. Her work also appears in the anthology *Stories of Strength*, benefiting the victims of Hurricane Katrina.

She lives and works in Los Angeles.

For information about Alyson's personal appearances and online workshops, join her email list at http://www.WakeUptoYourStories.com.